GENTLE STRETCHING EXERCISE FOR SENIORS OVER 60

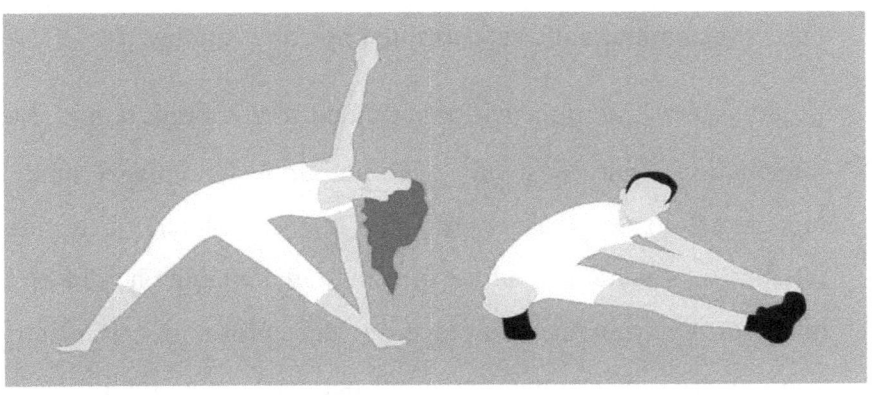

A Journey to Renewed Vitality Gentle Stretching for Vibrant Seniors

BERNARD D NELSON

Copyright © 2024 by Bernard D. Nelson

All rights reserved. No part of this publication may be reproduced, distributed, or transmitted in any form or by any means, including photocopying, recording, or other electronic or mechanical methods, without the prior written permission of the publisher, except in the case of brief quotations embodied in critical reviews and certain other noncommercial uses permitted by copyright law.

Disclaimer: The information provided in this book is for general informational purposes only. The author and publisher make no representations or warranties about the completeness, accuracy, reliability, or suitability of the information contained herein for any purpose. Any reliance you place on such information is strictly at your own risk. The author and publisher disclaim all liability arising from your use of or reliance on this book.

Trademark Acknowledgments: All product names, logos, and brands mentioned in this book are the property of their respective owners. Reference to any specific commercial product, process, or service does not constitute or imply endorsement, recommendation, or favoring by the author or publisher.

TABLE OF CONTENT

INTRODUCTION _____ 9

CHAPTER 1 _____ 13

    Introduction to Gentle Stretching _____ 13

    What is Gentle Stretching? _____ 13

    The Importance of Gentle Stretching for Seniors _____ 14

    The Benefits of Stretching for Seniors_____ 15

    Setting the Tone for the Book _____ 17

CHAPTER 2 _____ 19

    Understanding Aging and Flexibility _____ 19

    How Aging Affects Flexibility and Mobility_____ 20

    Common Issues and Challenges _____ 21

    The Importance of Maintaining Flexibility _____ 22

CHAPTER 3 _____ 25

    Getting Started Safely _____ 25

    Guidance on Preparing for Stretching Exercises_____ 26

    techniques you can incorporate into your routine_____ 26

    Safety Precautions and Tips _____ 27

Addressing Concerns or Hesitations _____ 29

CHAPTER 4 _____ 31

Essential Stretching Techniques _____ 31

Static Stretches _____ 32

Dynamic Stretches _____ 34

Proprioceptive Neuromuscular Facilitation (PNF) Stretches _____ 35

Step-by-Step Instructions and Illustrations _____ 36

_____ 37

CHAPTER 5 _____ 37

Full-Body Stretching Routine _____ 37

Upper Body Stretches _____ 38

Lower Body Stretches _____ 39

Core Stretches _____ 40

Modifications for Different Fitness Levels _____ 42

CHAPTER 6 _____ 43

Specialized Stretching Exercises _____ 43

Addressing Back Pain _____ 44

Addressing Arthritis _____ 45

Addressing Balance Issues _____ 46

CHAPTER 7 — 49

- Incorporating Stretching into Daily Life — 49
- The Importance of Consistency and Frequency — 49
- Practical Tips for Integrating Stretching into Daily Activities — 50
- Creating a Supportive Environment for Regular Stretching Practice — 52

CHAPTER 8 — 55

- Mindfulness and Relaxation Techniques — 55
- The Connection Between Stretching, Mindfulness, and Relaxation — 56
- Breathing Exercises — 56
- Meditation Techniques — 57
- Other Relaxation Practices — 59
- The Mental Health Benefits of Mindfulness in Stretching Routines — 60

CHAPTER 9 — 63

- Staying Motivated and Overcoming Challenges — 63
- Common Challenges Seniors May Face — 64
- Strategies for Staying Motivated and Overcoming Challenges — 65
- Success Stories and Testimonials — 66
- Conclusion — 68

CHAPTER 10 — 69

Maintaining Long-Term Flexibility and Health — 69

The Importance of Ongoing Maintenance and Progression — 70

Tips for Adapting the Stretching Routine — 70

The Role of Stretching in Supporting Overall Health and Independence — 72

CONCLUSION — 75

Embracing Your Journey to Vibrant Health — 75

Welcome to a journey of timeless vitality: 'Gentle Stretching for Seniors Over 60'— where every stretch unlocks the door to renewed flexibility, vitality, and a life lived

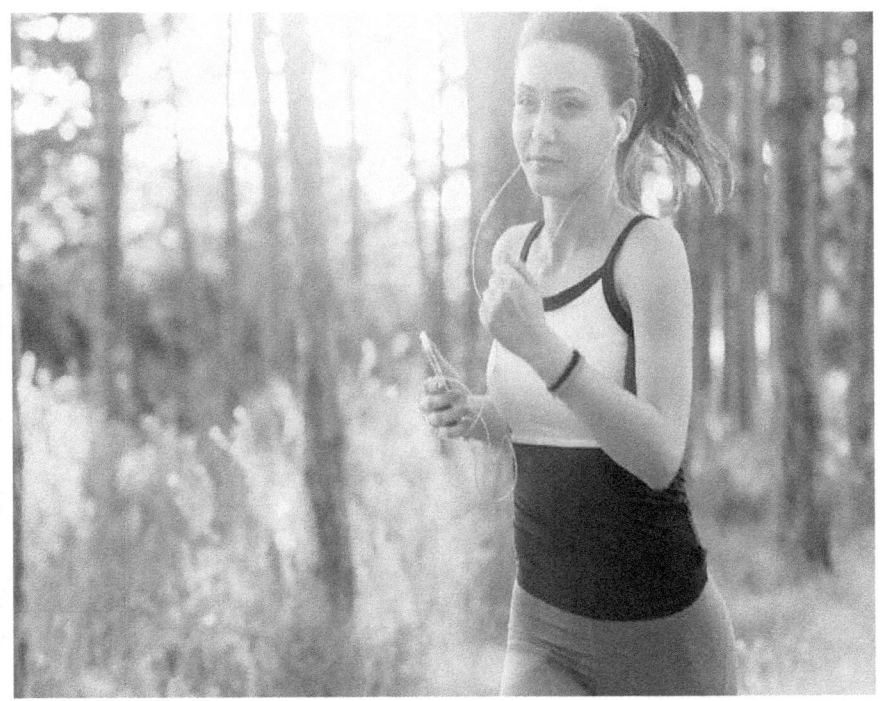

7 GENTLE STRETCHING EXERCISE FOR SENIORS OVER 60

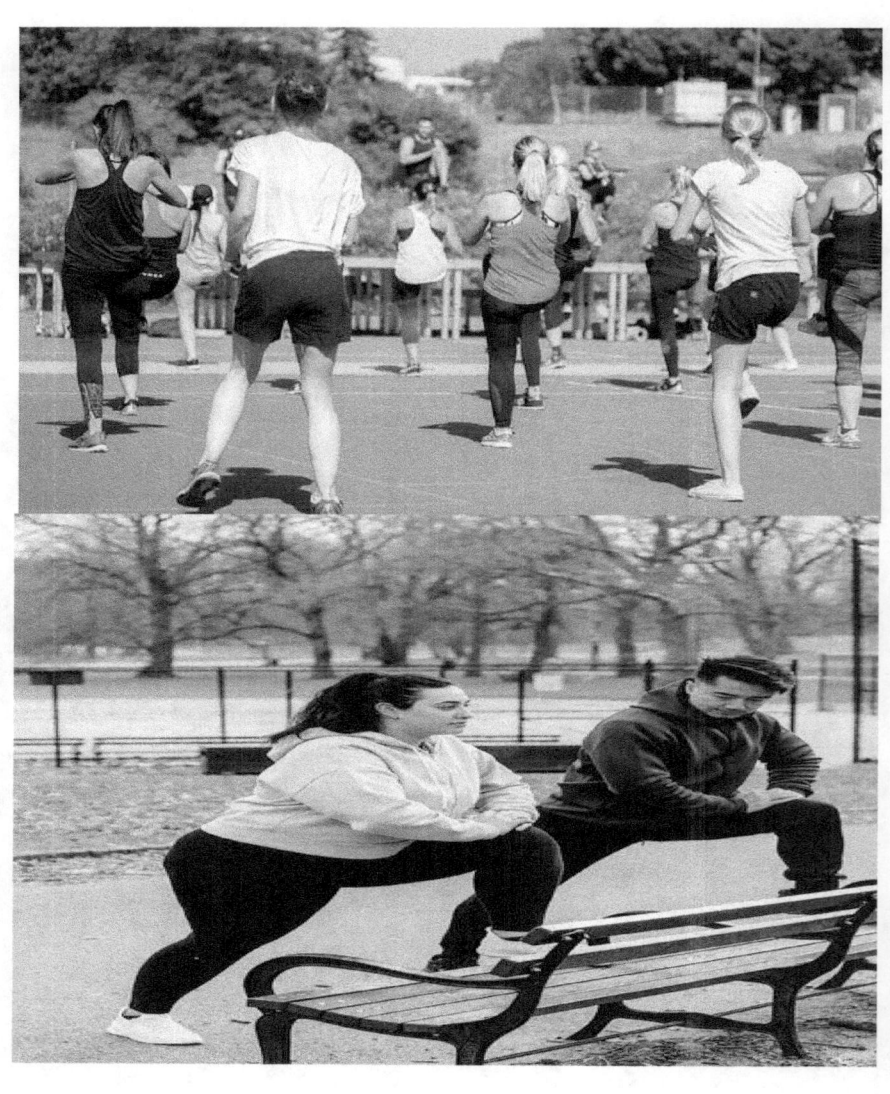

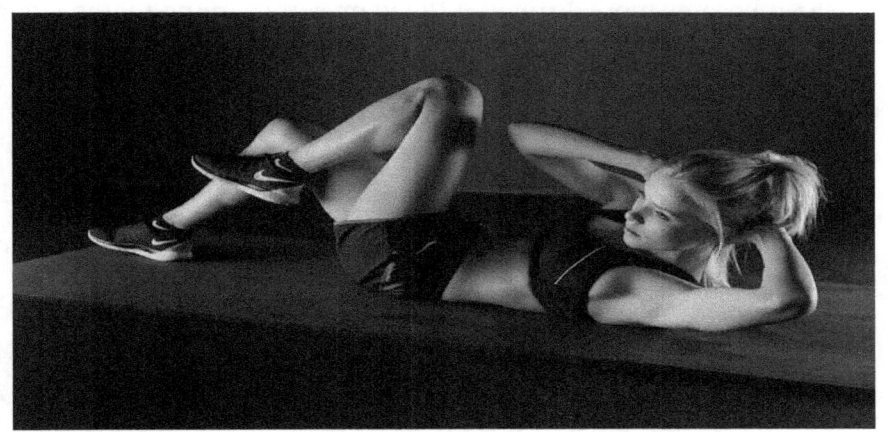

INTRODUCTION

As I sit in my favorite chair by the window, watching the world go by, I can't help but reflect on the journey that led me here. My name is Serah, and I'm a proud grandmother of three beautiful grandchildren. At sixty-five years old, I've seen my fair share of life's ups and downs. But today, as I look back, I realize that one of the most transformative experiences of my life began with a simple act—gentle stretching.

Growing older brings its own set of challenges. I remember the days when I could leap out of bed without a second thought, ready to tackle whatever the day brought my way. But as the years passed, I began to feel the effects of aging creeping in. My joints were stiffer, my muscles tighter, and simple tasks like bending down to tie my shoes became more difficult. I found myself yearning for the vitality and flexibility of my youth.

It was during one of my regular visits to the community center that I stumbled upon a flyer for a gentle stretching class specifically designed for seniors. Intrigued, I decided to give it a try. Little did I know that this decision would mark the beginning of a remarkable journey toward improved health, mobility, and a newfound sense of well-being.

In the beginning, I'll admit I was a bit skeptical. Stretching? Wasn't that something only athletes did before a workout? But as I settled into the class and began to follow along with the instructor's gentle movements, I felt a sense of relaxation wash over me. For the first time in years, I allowed myself to let go of the tension that had been building up in my body.

As the weeks went by, I started to notice subtle changes taking place within me. My muscles felt looser, my joints more flexible. Simple tasks like reaching for a high shelf or bending down to pick up a fallen object no longer felt like Herculean feats. But perhaps even more importantly, I found myself feeling more alive, more present in my own body.

It wasn't long before I began to explore stretching on my own outside of class. Armed with the knowledge I had gained from my instructor and fueled by a newfound sense of curiosity, I started to incorporate gentle stretching into my daily routine. Whether it was a few minutes of stretching before getting out of bed in the morning or a quick stretch break during a long day at work, I found that even the smallest gestures made a world of difference.

But the true power of gentle stretching revealed itself to me one sunny afternoon as I played with my grandchildren in the park. As I chased them around the playground, I couldn't help but marvel at the agility and boundless energy they possessed. But amidst the laughter and excitement, I also felt a twinge of sadness. Would I be able to keep up with them as they grew older? Would I be able to continue being the active, engaged grandmother they deserved?

It was in that moment that I made a promise to myself—to prioritize my health and well-being so that I could continue to be the best grandmother I could be. And so, my journey with gentle stretching took on a new sense of purpose. No longer was it simply about improving my own mobility and flexibility—it was about reclaiming my vitality and ensuring that I could continue to live life to the fullest, for myself and for those I loved.

And so, dear reader, it is with great joy and gratitude that I invite you to join me on this journey. In the pages that follow, you'll discover a treasure trove of gentle stretching exercises specifically tailored for seniors like us. Whether you're looking to alleviate joint pain, improve your balance, or simply reconnect with your body, you'll find practical tips, step-by-step instructions, and inspiring anecdotes to guide you every step of the way.

So let's embark on this adventure together, dear friend. Let's embrace the power of gentle stretching and unlock the full potential of our bodies and minds. After all, age is just a number—and with the right mindset and a willingness to try something new, anything is possible.

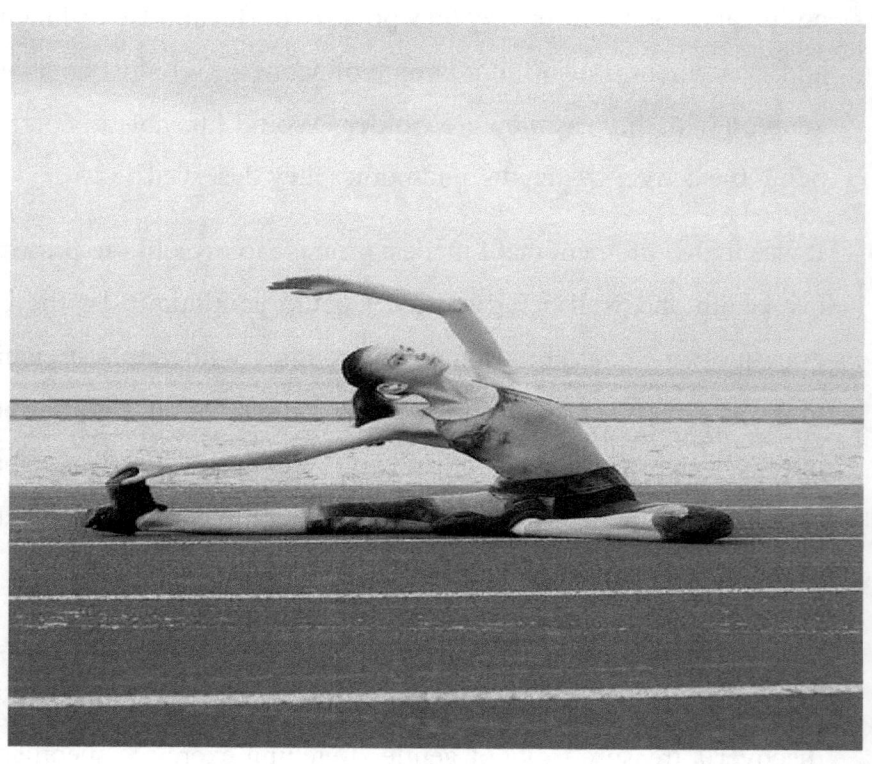

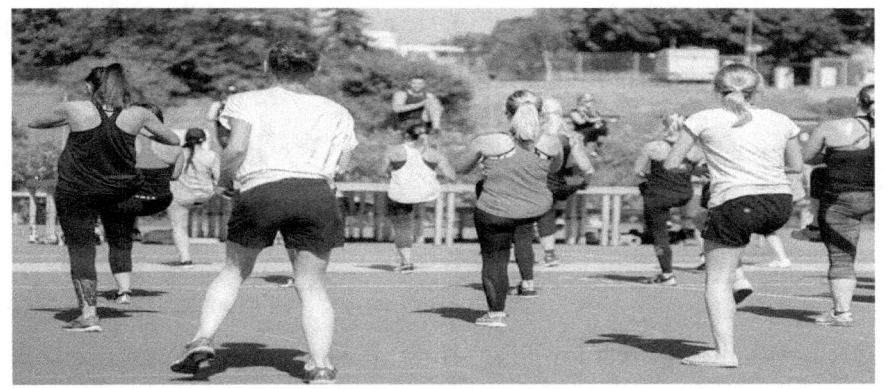

CHAPTER 1

Introduction to Gentle Stretching

Welcome to the beginning of your journey towards improved flexibility, mobility, and overall well-being through gentle stretching. In this chapter, we'll explore the definition and importance of gentle stretching for seniors, uncover the myriad benefits it offers, and set the tone for the rest of the book as your guide to safe and effective stretching exercises.

What is Gentle Stretching?

Gentle stretching involves moving your body in a slow, deliberate manner to lengthen and elongate your muscles gradually. Unlike more vigorous forms of exercise, such as weightlifting or high-intensity interval training, gentle stretching focuses on improving flexibility and mobility without putting undue stress on your joints or muscles. It's about listening to your body, respecting its limits, and honoring its unique needs as you move through each stretch.

The Importance of Gentle Stretching for Seniors

As we age, our bodies undergo a multitude of changes that can affect our flexibility and mobility. Joints may become stiffer, muscles may lose elasticity, and range of motion may decrease. Left unchecked, these changes can lead to increased risk of injury, decreased independence, and diminished quality of life. That's where gentle stretching comes in.

By incorporating gentle stretching into your daily routine, you can counteract the effects of aging and maintain or even improve your flexibility and mobility over time. Stretching helps to keep your muscles and joints supple, reducing stiffness and promoting better movement patterns. It can also improve circulation, enhance posture, and alleviate common aches and pains associated with aging.

But perhaps even more importantly, gentle stretching can have a profound impact on your overall well-being. It provides an opportunity to slow down, connect with your body, and cultivate a sense of mindfulness and presence in the moment. As you move through each stretch with intention and awareness, you'll not only improve your physical health but also nurture your mental and emotional health, reducing stress and promoting relaxation.

The Benefits of Stretching for Seniors

The benefits of gentle stretching for seniors are vast and varied, encompassing both physical and mental aspects of health and well-being. Here are just a few of the ways in which regular stretching can enhance your life:

1. Improved Flexibility: Stretching helps to lengthen and loosen tight muscles, allowing you to move more freely and with greater ease. Increased flexibility can make everyday activities such as bending,reaching, and twisting feel more comfortable and effortless.
2. Enhanced Mobility: By improving flexibility and range of motion, stretching can help you maintain or regain the ability to perform daily tasks independently, such as getting in and out of chairs, climbing stairs, and reaching for items on high shelves.
3. Reduced Risk of Injury: Flexible muscles and joints are less prone to strain and injury during physical activity. By regularly stretching, you can help prevent falls, strains, and other accidents that can result from stiffness or limited mobility.

4. **Better Posture:** Stretching exercises that target the muscles of the back, shoulders, and hips can help correct imbalances and alignment issues that contribute to poor posture. By standing taller and straighter, you'll not only look more confident but also reduce strain on your spine and joints.

5. **Pain Relief:** Stretching can help alleviate common aches and pains associated with aging, such as back pain, arthritis, and stiffness. By gently elongating tight muscles and releasing tension, you can experience relief from discomfort and enjoy greater comfort and ease in your daily life.

6. **Improved Circulation:** Stretching increases blood flow to the muscles, which can help improve circulation and promote healing. Better circulation means more oxygen and nutrients reaching your tissues, leading to faster recovery from injuries and enhanced overall health.

7. **Stress Reduction:** Engaging in gentle stretching can have a calming effect on the nervous system, reducing levels of stress hormones such as cortisol and promoting a sense of relaxation and well-being. By taking time to slow down and breathe deeply, you can release tension and find peace amidst the busyness of life.

Setting the Tone for the Book

As you embark on this journey of self-discovery and self-care, it's important to approach gentle stretching with an open mind and a spirit of curiosity. This book is not just a manual of exercises but a roadmap to a healthier, happier you. Throughout the pages that follow, you'll find a wealth of practical tips, step-by-step instructions, and inspiring stories to guide you on your stretching journey.

But remember, the most important thing is to listen to your body and honor its needs. If a stretch feels uncomfortable or painful, back off and try a gentler variation. And always consult with your healthcare provider before beginning any new exercise program, especially if you have pre-existing health conditions or concerns.

So let's dive in together, dear reader, and explore the transformative power of gentle stretching. Whether you're looking to improve your flexibility, reduce pain, or simply reconnect with your body, this book is here to support you every step of the way. Get ready to stretch, strengthen, and soar into a brighter, more vibrant future!

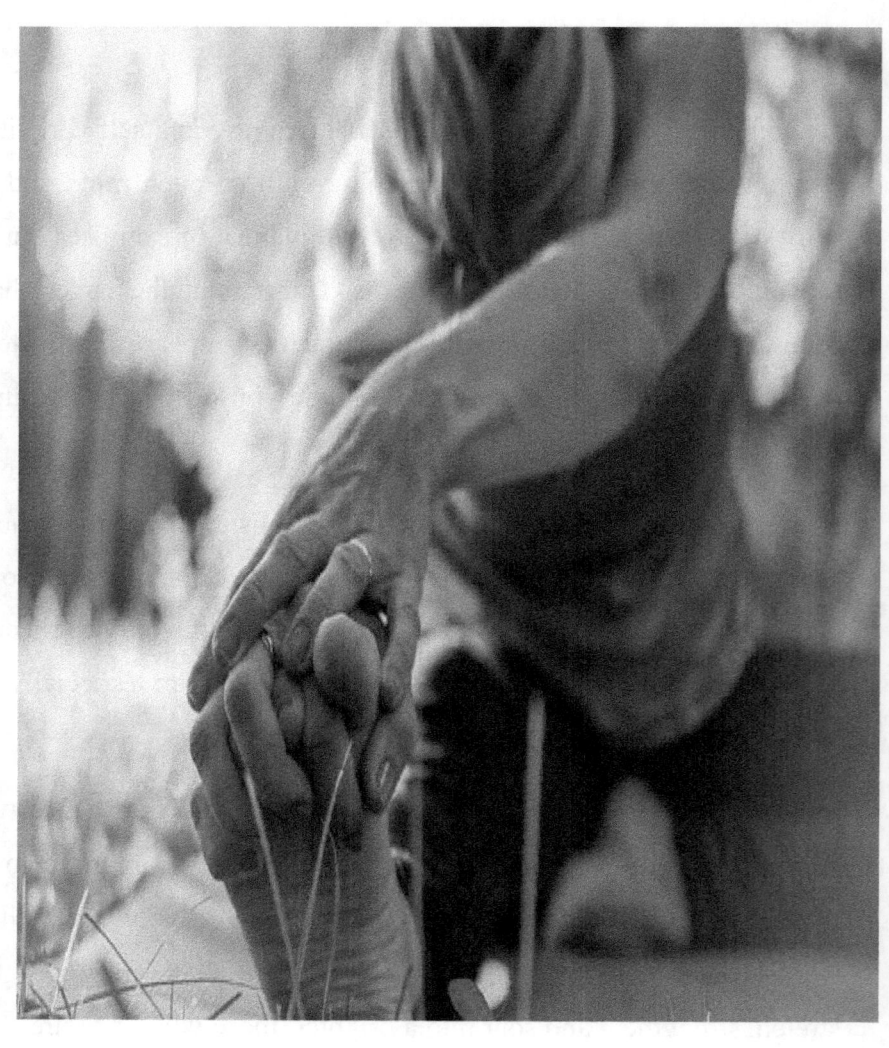

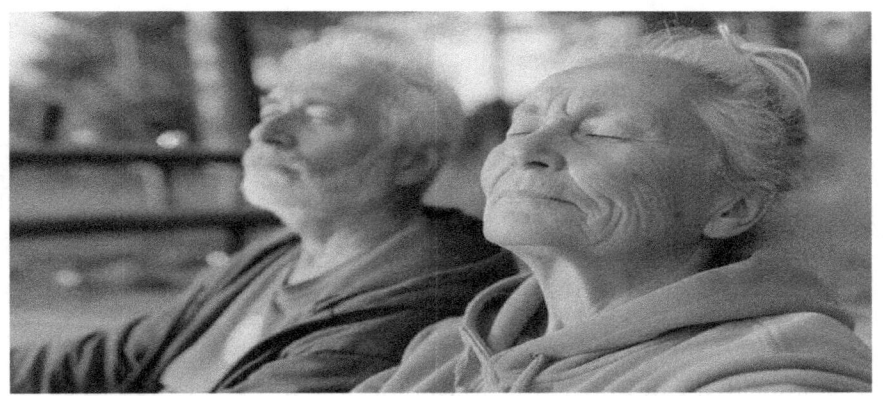

CHAPTER 2

Understanding Aging and Flexibility

Welcome to Chapter 2. In this chapter, we'll explore the intricate relationship between aging and flexibility, uncovering the ways in which the passage of time can impact our bodies and mobility. We'll discuss common issues such as joint stiffness, decreased muscle mass, and reduced range of motion, and emphasize the importance of maintaining flexibility as we age. By understanding these factors, you'll gain valuable insights into how gentle stretching can help counteract the effects of aging and support your overall health and well-being.

How Aging Affects Flexibility and Mobility

As we journey through life, our bodies undergo a series of changes that can affect our flexibility and mobility. One of the most significant factors contributing to these changes is the natural aging process. As we age, several physiological changes occur within our bodies that can impact our musculoskeletal system:

1. Loss of Elasticity: With age, the connective tissues in our muscles and tendons become less elastic, leading to decreased flexibility and range of motion. This loss of elasticity can make it more difficult to perform simple tasks such as bending, reaching, and twisting.
2. Decreased Muscle Mass: As we get older, we tend to lose muscle mass and strength—a phenomenon known as sarcopenia. This loss of muscle mass can further contribute to decreased flexibility and mobility, making it harder to move with ease and perform activities of daily living.
3. Joint Changes: The cartilage that cushions our joints may begin to deteriorate over time, leading to stiffness, pain, and reduced mobility. Conditions such as osteoarthritis can exacerbate these changes, further limiting our ability to move comfortably and freely.

4. **Postural Changes:** As we age, changes in posture and alignment can also affect our flexibility and mobility. Poor posture, weakened muscles, and imbalanced movement patterns can lead to decreased range of motion and increased risk of injury.

While these changes are a natural part of the aging process, they don't have to be inevitable. By incorporating gentle stretching into your daily routine, you can help counteract the effects of aging and maintain or even improve your flexibility and mobility over time.

Common Issues and Challenges

There are several common issues and challenges that seniors may face when it comes to flexibility and mobility. Understanding these challenges can help you better navigate your stretching journey and address any obstacles that may arise.

1. **Joint Stiffness:** Joint stiffness is a common complaint among seniors, especially in the morning or after periods of inactivity. Stiffness can make it difficult to move freely and may contribute to decreased range of motion and increased risk of injury.
2. **Decreased Range of Motion:** As we age, our range of motion—the distance through which we can move a joint—may become more limited. This can affect our ability to

perform everyday tasks such as bending, reaching, and turning, and may contribute to feelings of frustration or immobility.

3. Muscle Tightness: Tight muscles are another common issue among seniors, often resulting from a combination of factors such as inactivity, poor posture, and decreased flexibility. Muscle tightness can lead to discomfort, pain, and reduced mobility, making it harder to move with ease and grace.

5. Balance and Stability: Maintaining balance and stability becomes increasingly important as we age, as falls and injuries become more common. Poor balance can be caused by a variety of factors, including muscle weakness, joint stiffness, and changes in proprioception (the body's sense of its own position in space).

The Importance of Maintaining Flexibility

In the face of these challenges, maintaining flexibility becomes paramount for seniors seeking to preserve their mobility and independence. Flexibility is the key to maintaining a full range of motion in your joints, allowing you to move more freely and comfortably throughout your day. By incorporating gentle stretching into your routine, you can help counteract the effects of aging and promote better flexibility and mobility for years to come.

But the benefits of maintaining flexibility extend beyond just physical health. Flexibility is also closely linked to mental and emotional well-being, providing a sense of freedom, vitality, and empowerment. By cultivating flexibility in both body and mind, you can approach life's challenges with greater ease and resilience, embracing new opportunities and experiences with open arms.

In the next chapters, we'll explore practical strategies for improving flexibility through gentle stretching exercises specifically tailored for seniors. Whether you're looking to alleviate joint stiffness, increase range of motion, or simply enjoy greater freedom of movement, you'll find valuable insights and guidance to support you on your journey to improved flexibility and mobility.

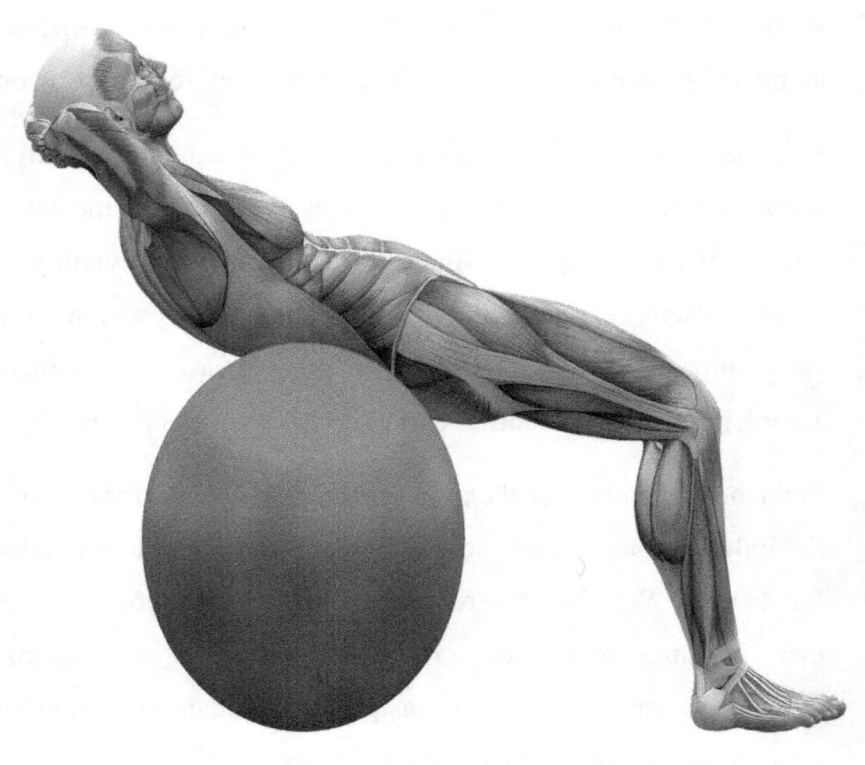

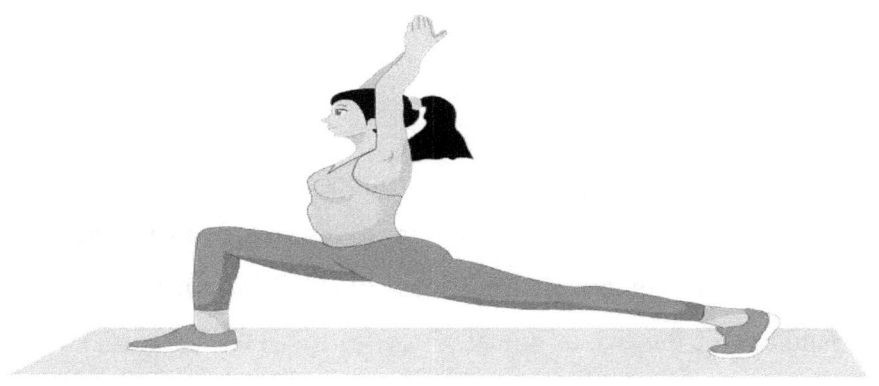

CHAPTER 3

Getting Started Safely

Welcome to Chapter 3. In this chapter, we'll explore the importance of getting started safely on your stretching journey. We'll provide guidance on preparing for stretching exercises, including warm-up techniques to help you ease into your routine. We'll also discuss safety precautions and tips for avoiding injury, as well as address any concerns or hesitations you may have about starting a stretching routine. By prioritizing safety and taking a gradual approach, you'll set yourself up for success and enjoy all the benefits that gentle stretching has to offer.

Guidance on Preparing for Stretching Exercises

Before you begin your stretching routine, it's important to take some time to prepare your body and mind. This includes warming up your muscles and joints to help increase blood flow, improve flexibility, and reduce the risk of injury.

Here are some gentle warm-up

techniques you can incorporate into your routine

1. Dynamic Movements: Start by performing gentle, dynamic movements to gradually increase your heart rate and warm up your muscles. This can include movements such as arm circles, leg swings, and gentle torso twists.
2. Cardiovascular Exercise: If possible, engage in a few minutes of light cardiovascular exercise, such as walking or cycling, to further increase blood flow and prepare your body for stretching.
3. Joint Mobilization: Spend some time focusing on mobilizing your joints through gentle movements such as ankle circles, wrist circles, and neck rolls. This can help lubricate the joints and improve range of motion.

4. **Deep Breathing:** Incorporate deep breathing exercises into your warm-up routine to help relax your body and calm your mind. Take slow, deep breaths in through your nose, filling your lungs with air, and exhale slowly through your mouth.

By taking the time to properly warm up your body before stretching, you'll help reduce the risk of injury and ensure that you get the most out of your stretching routine.

Safety Precautions and Tips

Safety should always be your top priority when engaging in any form of physical activity, including stretching. Here are some important safety precautions and tips to keep in mind:

1. **Listen to Your Body:** Pay attention to how your body feels during stretching exercises. If you experience any pain or discomfort, ease off and try a gentler variation of the stretch. Never force your body into a stretch beyond its limits.

2. **Start Slowly:** If you're new to stretching or haven't exercised in a while, start slowly and gradually increase the intensity and duration of your stretches over time. Rome wasn't built in a day, and neither is flexibility.

3. **Use Props and Support:** If you have trouble reaching certain areas or maintaining proper alignment during stretches, use props such as yoga blocks, straps, or pillows to provide support and assistance.

4. **Stay Hydrated:** Drink plenty of water before, during, and after your stretching routine to stay hydrated and help prevent muscle cramps and fatigue.

6. **Avoid Bouncing:** Avoid bouncing or jerking movements during stretches, as this can strain your muscles and increase the risk of injury. Instead, focus on slow, controlled movements and gentle, sustained stretches.

7. **Be Mindful of Your Environment:** Choose a safe and comfortable environment for stretching, free from obstacles or hazards that could cause accidents or falls.

8. **Consult with Your Healthcare Provider:** If you have any pre-existing health conditions or concerns, or if you're unsure whether stretching is safe for you, consult with your healthcare provider before beginning a new stretching routine.

By following these safety precautions and tips, you can minimize the risk of injury and ensure a safe and enjoyable stretching experience.

Addressing Concerns or Hesitations

It's natural to have concerns or hesitations about starting a stretching routine, especially if you're unfamiliar with the practice or have had negative experiences with exercise in the past. Here are some common concerns that seniors may have about stretching, along with strategies for addressing them;

1. Fear of Injury: Many seniors worry about injuring themselves while stretching, particularly if they have pre-existing health conditions or limited mobility. By starting slowly, listening to your body, and following proper technique, you can minimize the risk of injury and gradually build confidence in your stretching abilities.

2. Feeling Intimidated: Some seniors may feel intimidated by the idea of starting a stretching routine, especially if they're unfamiliar with the exercises or don't consider themselves to be "athletic." Remember that stretching is for everyone, regardless of age, fitness level, or experience. Start where you are, and progress at your own pace.

3. Lack of Time: Many seniors lead busy lives and may struggle to find the time to incorporate stretching into their daily routine. Remember that even a few minutes of stretching each day can make a big difference in your flexibility and mobility over time. Consider incorporating

stretches into activities you already do, such as watching TV or reading a book.

4. **Concerns About Effectiveness:** Some seniors may wonder whether stretching is truly effective or if it's just a waste of time. Research has shown that regular stretching can lead to significant improvements in flexibility, mobility, and overall well-being, even in older adults. Trust in the process and give yourself time to experience the benefits for yourself.

By addressing these concerns and hesitations head-on, you can overcome barriers to starting a stretching routine and embark on your journey to improved flexibility and mobility with confidence and enthusiasm.

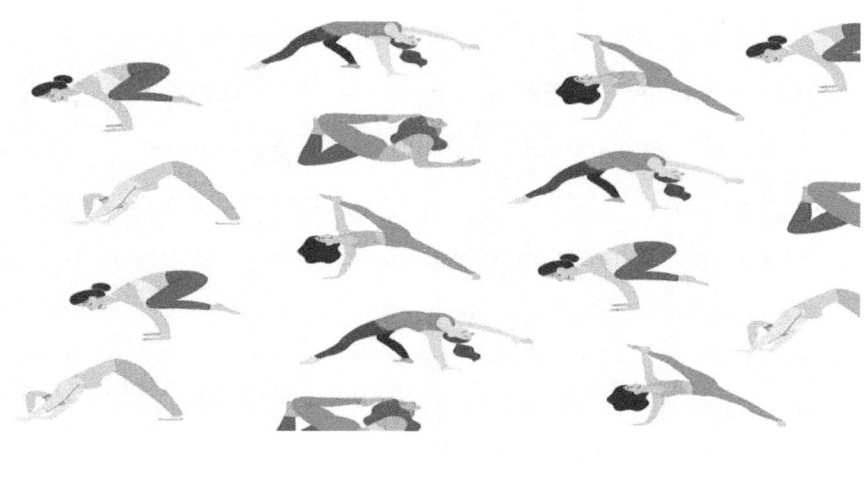

CHAPTER 4

Essential Stretching Techniques

Welcome to Chapter 4. In this chapter, we'll introduce you to a variety of essential stretching techniques specifically designed for seniors. Whether you're new to stretching or looking to expand your repertoire, you'll find a range of gentle and effective stretches to help improve flexibility, mobility, and overall well-being. We'll cover static stretches, dynamic stretches, and proprioceptive neuromuscular facilitation (PNF) stretches, providing step-by-step instructions and illustrations for each technique to ensure proper form and safety.

Static Stretches

Static stretches involve holding a specific position for a period of time to elongate and relax the muscles. These stretches are excellent for improving flexibility and range of motion, as well as relieving tension and promoting relaxation. Here are some essential static stretches for seniors:

1. Neck Stretch: **Sit or stand tall with your shoulders relaxed. Gently tilt your head to one side, bringing your ear towards your shoulder until you feel a stretch along the side of your neck. Hold for 15-30 seconds, then switch sides.**

2. Shoulder Stretch: **Bring one arm across your body, using your other hand to gently press the arm towards your chest until you feel a stretch in your shoulder and upper back. Hold for 15-30 seconds, then switch sides.**

3. Chest Opener: **Stand tall with your feet hip-width apart. Clasp your hands behind your back and gently straighten your arms, lifting your chest towards the ceiling. Hold for 15-30 seconds, focusing on opening up the chest and shoulders.**

4. Hamstring Stretch: **Sit on the floor with one leg extended and the other bent. Reach towards your toes with both hands, keeping your back straight and chest lifted. Hold for 15-30 seconds, then switch legs.**

5. Calf Stretch: Stand facing a wall with your hands resting against it for support. Step one foot back and press the heel into the ground, feeling a stretch in the calf of the back leg. Hold for 15-30 seconds, then switch legs.

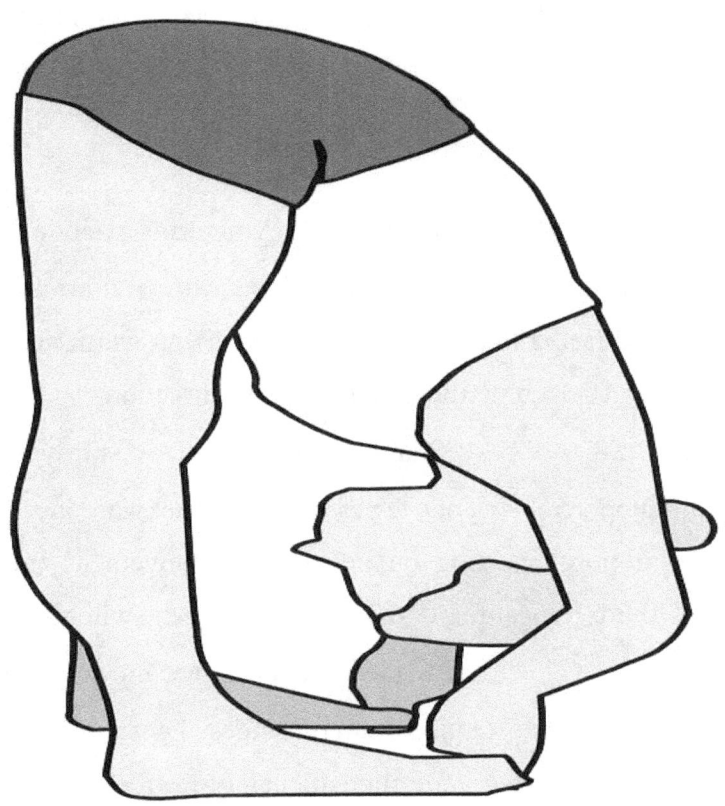

Dynamic Stretches

Dynamic stretches involve moving your body through a full range of motion in a controlled manner to warm up the muscles and increase blood flow. These stretches are great for improving flexibility, mobility, and circulation, especially before engaging in more vigorous physical activity.

Here are some essential dynamic stretches for seniors:

1. Arm Circles: **Stand tall with your arms extended out to the sides. Begin making small circles with your arms, gradually increasing the size of the circles as you warm up. Continue for 10-15 repetitions, then reverse direction.**
2. Leg Swings: **Stand facing a wall or sturdy object for support. Swing one leg forward and backward in a controlled motion, focusing on keeping the movement smooth and fluid. Repeat for 10-15 repetitions, then switch legs.**
3. Torso Twists: **Stand with your feet hip-width apart and your arms extended out to the sides. Twist your torso to one side, reaching your opposite hand towards the back. Return to center and repeat on the other side. Continue for 10-15 repetitions.**

4. Hip Circles: Stand tall with your hands on your hips. Circle your hips in a clockwise motion, focusing on moving smoothly and without strain. Repeat for 10-15 repetitions, then reverse direction.

Proprioceptive Neuromuscular Facilitation (PNF) Stretches

PNF stretches involve alternating between contracting and relaxing the muscles to enhance flexibility and range of motion. These stretches are often done with a partner but can also be modified for solo practice. Here are some essential PNF stretches for seniors:

1. Hamstring PNF Stretch: Lie on your back with one leg extended and the other bent. Have a partner gently press your extended leg towards your chest as you resist the movement with your own strength. Hold for a few seconds, then relax and deepen the stretch. Repeat 2-3 times, then switch legs.
2. Shoulder PNF Stretch: Sit or stand with one arm extended out to the side at shoulder height. Have a partner gently push your arm down towards the floor as you resist the movement with your own strength. Hold for a few seconds, then relax and deepen the stretch. Repeat 2-3 times, then switch arms.

Step-by-Step Instructions and Illustrations

Throughout this chapter, you'll find detailed step-by-step instructions and illustrations for each stretching technique to help you perform the exercises safely and effectively. These visual aids will guide you through proper form and alignment, ensuring that you get the most out of your stretching routine while minimizing the risk of injury.

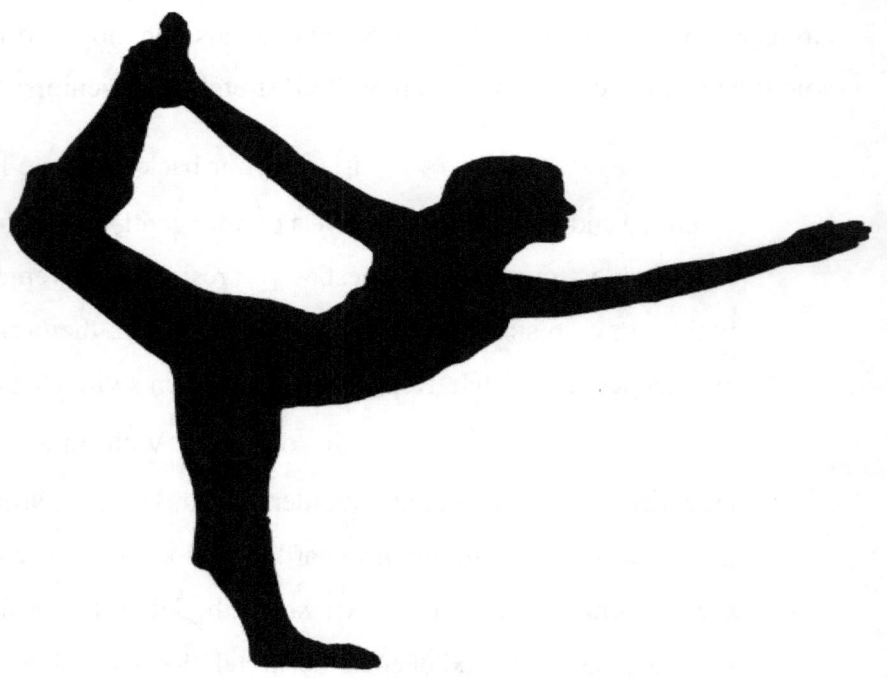

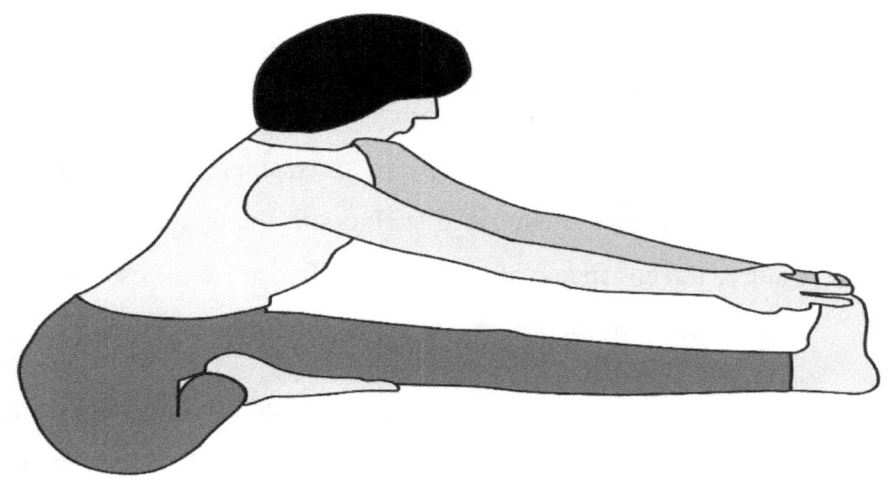

CHAPTER 5

Full-Body Stretching Routine

Welcome to Chapter 5 In this chapter, we'll present a comprehensive full-body stretching routine specifically designed to promote flexibility, mobility, and overall well-being in seniors. We'll divide the routine into sections targeting different muscle groups, including the upper body, lower body, and core, and provide modifications for different fitness levels and abilities. Whether you're a beginner or an experienced stretcher, you'll find valuable exercises to help you feel more limber, relaxed, and rejuvenated.

Upper Body Stretches

We'll start our full-body stretching routine by focusing on the upper body, including the neck, shoulders, arms, and chest. These stretches can help alleviate tension and stiffness in the upper body, improve posture, and enhance range of motion. Here are some essential upper body stretches to incorporate into your routine:

1. Neck Stretch: Gently tilt your head to one side, bringing your ear towards your shoulder until you feel a stretch along the side of your neck. Hold for 15-30 seconds, then switch sides.

3. Shoulder Stretch: Bring one arm across your body and use your other hand to gently press the arm towards your chest until you feel a stretch in your shoulder and upper back. Hold for 15-30 seconds, then switch sides.

4. Triceps Stretch: Reach one arm overhead and bend the elbow, bringing your hand down towards your upper back. Use your other hand to gently press the elbow towards the center of your back until you feel a stretch in the back of your arm. Hold for 15-30 seconds, then switch arms.

5. Chest Opener: Clasp your hands behind your back and gently straighten your arms, lifting your chest towards the ceiling. Hold for 15-30 seconds, focusing on opening up the chest and shoulders.

Lower Body Stretches

Next, we'll move on to stretches targeting the lower body, including the hips, thighs, calves, and feet. These stretches can help improve flexibility, reduce stiffness, and alleviate discomfort in the lower body. Here are some essential lower body stretches to incorporate into your routine:

1. Hamstring Stretch: Sit on the floor with one leg extended and the other bent. Reach towards your toes with both hands, keeping your back straight and chest lifted. Hold for 15-30 seconds, then switch legs.
2. Quadriceps Stretch: Stand tall and bend one knee, bringing your heel towards your buttocks. Use your hand to gently pull the foot towards your glutes until you feel a stretch in the front of your thigh. Hold for 15-30 seconds, then switch legs.
3. Calf Stretch: Stand facing a wall with your hands resting against it for support. Step one foot back and press the heel into the ground, feeling a stretch in the calf of the back leg. Hold for 15-30 seconds, then switch legs.
4. Hip Flexor Stretch: Kneel on one knee with the other foot planted on the ground in front of you. Lean forward slightly, keeping your back straight, until you feel a stretch in the front of your hip. Hold for 15-30 seconds, then switch sides.

Core Stretches

Finally, we'll target the muscles of the core, including the abdominals, obliques, and lower back. These stretches can help improve posture, balance, and stability, as well as alleviate discomfort in the lower back.

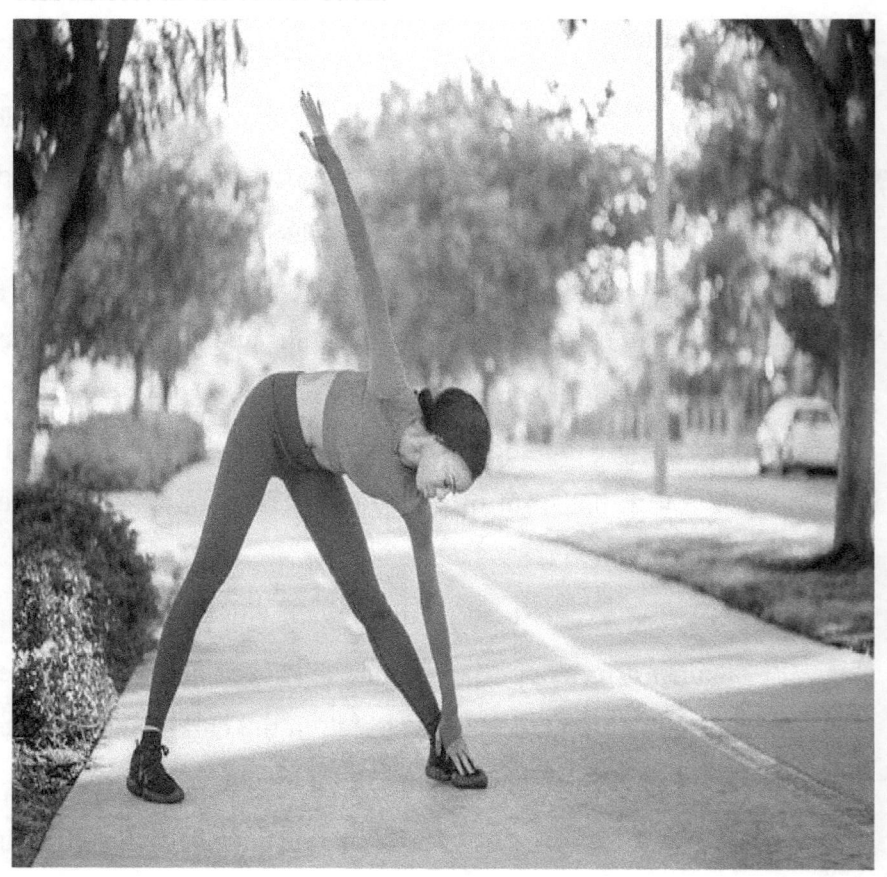

Here are some essential core stretches to incorporate into your routine:

1. **Cat-Cow Stretch:** Start on your hands and knees with your back flat and your wrists directly under your shoulders. Inhale as you arch your back, lifting your chest and tailbone towards the ceiling (cow pose). Exhale as you round your back, tucking your chin to your chest and drawing your belly button towards your spine (cat pose). Repeat for 10-15 repetitions, moving with your breath.
2. **Seated Forward Fold:** Sit on the floor with your legs extended in front of you. Hinge at the hips and fold forward, reaching towards your toes with your hands. Keep your back straight and chest lifted as you lengthen through the spine. Hold for 15-30 seconds, focusing on stretching the muscles of the lower back and hamstrings.
3. **Side Stretch:** Sit on the floor with your legs extended to one side and your hands on the ground for support. Reach one arm overhead and lean towards the opposite side, feeling a stretch along the side of your torso. Hold for 15-30 seconds, then switch sides.

Modifications for Different Fitness Levels

It's important to remember that everyone's body is different, and what works for one person may not work for another. That's why we've included modifications for each stretch to accommodate different fitness levels and abilities. If a stretch feels too intense, back off and try a gentler variation. And if you're feeling up for a challenge, you can always deepen the stretch or hold it for longer to increase the intensity.

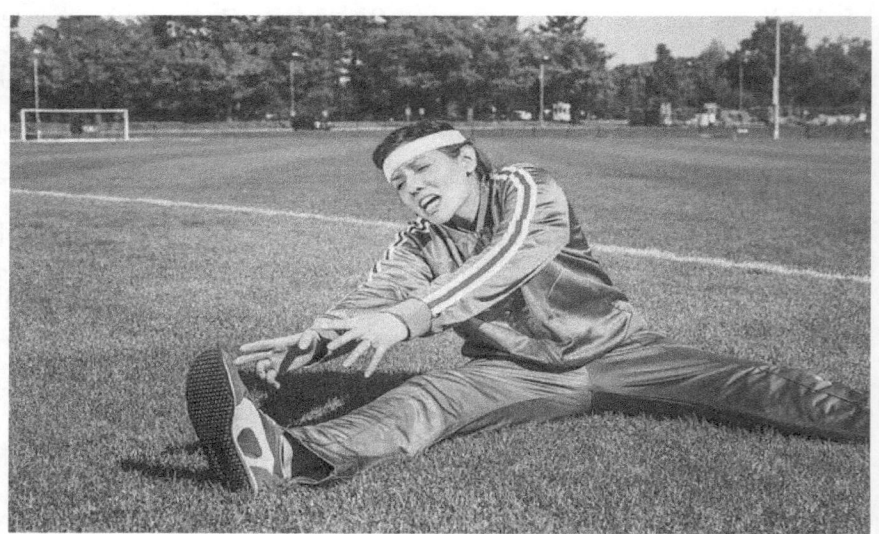

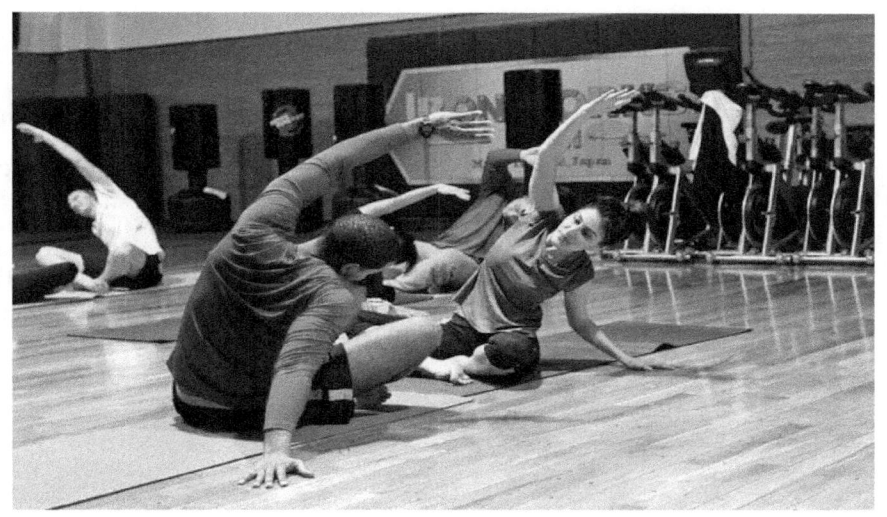

CHAPTER 6

Specialized Stretching Exercises

Welcome to Chapter 6 In this chapter, we'll address specific areas of concern for seniors, such as back pain, arthritis, and balance issues. We'll provide targeted stretching exercises and modifications tailored to these conditions, along with tips for managing discomfort and improving mobility. Whether you're dealing with chronic pain or seeking to enhance your balance and stability, you'll find valuable insights and guidance to help you feel stronger, more flexible, and more resilient.

Addressing Back Pain

Back pain is a common complaint among seniors, often resulting from a combination of factors such as poor posture, muscle imbalances, and age-related changes in the spine. Stretching exercises can help alleviate back pain by relieving tension in the muscles, improving flexibility, and promoting better alignment. Here are some specialized stretching exercises for addressing back pain:

1. Child's Pose: Start on your hands and knees with your toes touching and knees spread wide apart. Sit back on your heels and reach your arms forward, lowering your chest towards the floor. Hold for 15-30 seconds, feeling a stretch in your back and hips.

2. Cat-Cow Stretch: Start on your hands and knees with your back flat. Inhale as you arch your back, lifting your chest and tailbone towards the ceiling (cow pose). Exhale as you round your back, tucking your chin to your chest (cat pose). Repeat for 10-15 repetitions, moving with your breath.

3. Knee-to-Chest Stretch: Lie on your back with your knees bent and feet flat on the floor. Bring one knee towards your chest and grasp it with both hands, pulling it gently towards

your chest until you feel a stretch in your lower back. Hold for 15-30 seconds, then switch legs.

Addressing Arthritis

Arthritis is a common condition that causes inflammation and stiffness in the joints, leading to pain and reduced mobility. Stretching exercises can help improve joint mobility, reduce stiffness, and alleviate discomfort associated with arthritis.

Here are some specialized stretching exercises for addressing arthritis:

1. Wrist Flexor Stretch: Extend one arm in front of you with the palm facing down. Use your other hand to gently press the fingers towards the floor until you feel a stretch in your wrist and forearm. Hold for 15-30 seconds, then switch arms.
2. Hip Flexor Stretch: Kneel on one knee with the other foot planted on the ground in front of you. Lean forward slightly, keeping your back straight, until you feel a stretch in the front of your hip. Hold for 15-30 seconds, then switch sides.
3. Ankle Plantar Flexor Stretch: Sit on the floor with one leg extended in front of you and the other knee bent. Loop a towel or resistance band around the ball of your foot and gently pull it towards you, feeling a stretch in your calf and ankle. Hold for 15-30 seconds, then switch legs.

Addressing Balance Issues

Maintaining balance becomes increasingly important as we age, as falls and injuries become more common. Stretching exercises that target the muscles of the lower body, core, and proprioception (the body's sense of its own position in space) can help improve balance and stability.

Here are some specialized stretching exercises for addressing balance issues:

1. Single Leg Balance: Stand tall with your feet hip-width apart. Shift your weight onto one leg and lift the other leg off the ground, balancing on one foot. Hold for 15-30 seconds, then switch legs. For an added challenge, try closing your eyes or standing on a cushioned surface.

2. Tree Pose: Stand tall with your feet hip-width apart and arms by your sides. Shift your weight onto one leg and bend the other knee, placing the sole of your foot against the inner thigh or calf of the standing leg. Press your palms together at your chest and hold for 15-30 seconds, then switch legs.

3. Heel-to-Toe Walk: Stand with your feet in a straight line, with the heel of one foot touching the toes of the other. Take small steps forward, placing the heel of one foot directly in

front of the toes of the other. Walk in a straight line for 10-15 steps, focusing on maintaining balance and stability.

Tips for Managing Discomfort and Improving Mobility

In addition to incorporating stretching exercises into your routine, there are several other strategies you can use to manage discomfort and improve mobility:

1. Stay Hydrated: Drink plenty of water throughout the day to keep your joints lubricated and your muscles hydrated.
2. Use Heat and Cold Therapy: Applying heat packs or cold packs to sore or stiff joints can help reduce inflammation and alleviate pain.
3. Practice Mindfulness and Relaxation Techniques: Engage in activities such as deep breathing, meditation, or gentle yoga to reduce stress and promote relaxation, which can help alleviate tension and discomfort in the body.
4. Stay Active: Incorporate regular physical activity into your routine, such as walking, swimming, or cycling, to improve strength, flexibility, and overall mobility.
5. Listen to Your Body: Pay attention to how your body feels during stretching exercises, and adjust your routine accordingly. If a stretch feels uncomfortable or painful, back off and try a gentler variation.

By incorporating these specialized stretching exercises into your routine and following these tips for managing discomfort and improving mobility, you can enhance your overall quality of life and enjoy greater freedom of movement and vitality.

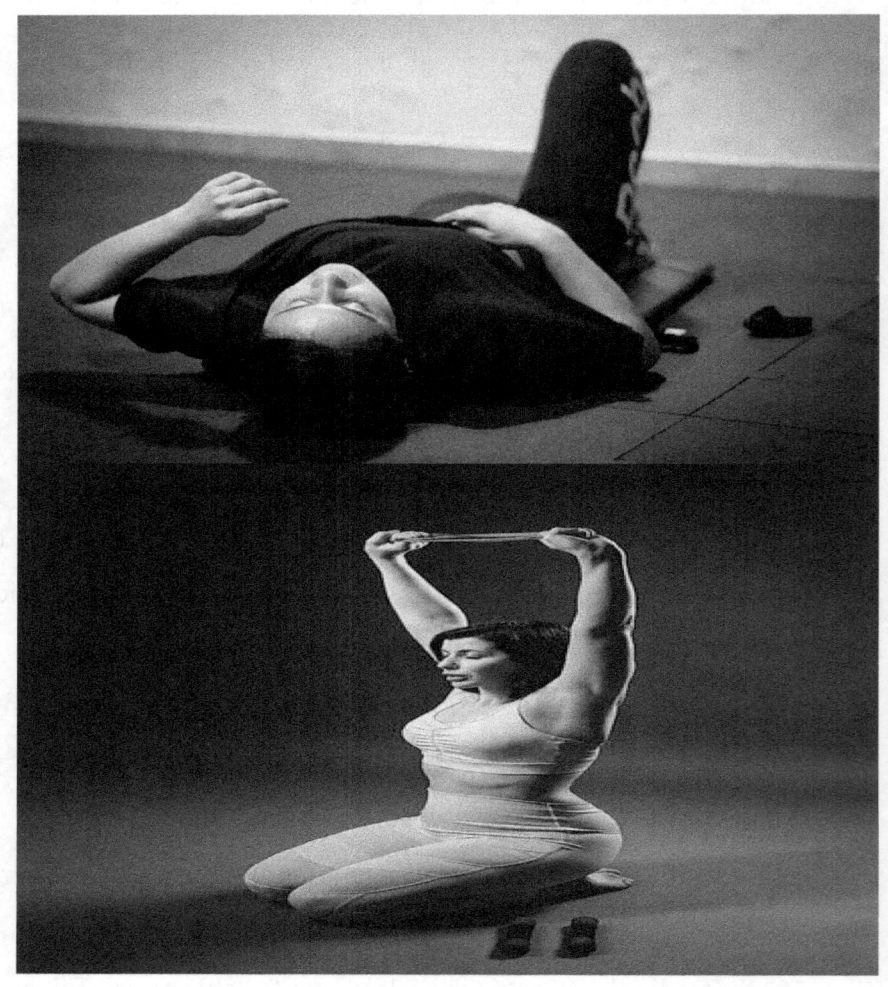

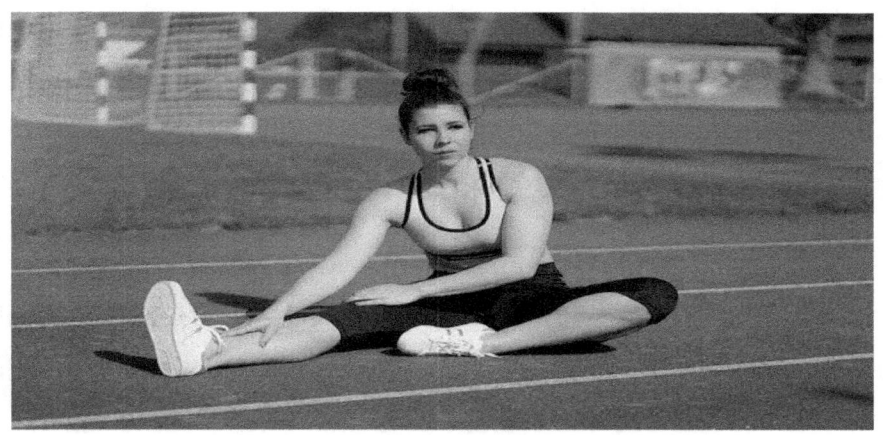

CHAPTER 7

Incorporating Stretching into Daily Life

Welcome to Chapter 7 In this chapter, we'll discuss the importance of consistency and frequency in a stretching routine and provide practical tips for integrating stretching exercises into your daily activities. We'll also offer suggestions for creating a supportive environment for regular stretching practice, so you can reap the full benefits of improved flexibility, mobility, and overall well-being in your everyday life.

The Importance of Consistency and Frequency

Consistency and frequency are key components of any successful stretching routine. Just like any other form of exercise, stretching requires regular practice to maintain and improve flexibility, mobility, and range of motion. By incorporating stretching into your daily routine, you'll gradually build flexibility and strength in your muscles and joints, making it easier to move with ease and grace.

Consistency is also important for preventing injury and maintaining the benefits of stretching over time. If you only stretch sporadically, you may not see significant improvements in flexibility or mobility, and you may be more prone to injury when you do engage in physical activity. By making stretching a regular part of your daily routine, you'll ensure that you continue to reap the rewards of improved flexibility and mobility for years to come.

Practical Tips for Integrating Stretching into Daily Activities

Integrating stretching exercises into your daily activities doesn't have to be complicated or time-consuming. With a little creativity and planning, you can incorporate stretching into your day in simple and convenient ways. Here are some practical tips to help you integrate stretching into your daily life:

1. Start Small: Begin by incorporating just a few minutes of stretching into your daily routine, such as stretching your arms and legs when you wake up in the morning or before you go to bed at night. As you become more comfortable

with stretching, you can gradually increase the duration and intensity of your routine.

2. Schedule Stretch Breaks: Set aside specific times throughout the day for short stretching breaks, such as mid-morning and mid-afternoon. Use these breaks as an opportunity to stretch your muscles and joints, relieve tension, and refresh your mind and body.

3. Combine Stretching with Other Activities: Look for opportunities to combine stretching with other activities you enjoy, such as watching TV, reading a book, or talking on the phone. Stretching while engaged in these activities can make the time pass more quickly and make stretching feel like less of a chore.

4. Incorporate Stretching into Your Workday: If you have a sedentary job that requires sitting for long periods, make an effort to incorporate stretching into your workday. Set a timer to remind yourself to stand up and stretch every hour, or perform seated stretches at your desk to relieve tension in your neck, shoulders, and back.

5. Make It a Family Affair: Get your family members or household members involved in stretching with you. Set aside time each day to stretch together as a family, or encourage your loved ones to join you for a post-dinner stretching session.

6. Use Everyday Objects as Props: Incorporate everyday objects such as chairs, walls, and countertops into your stretching routine to provide support and assistance. For example, you can use a chair for seated hamstring stretches or a wall for calf stretches.

Creating a Supportive Environment for Regular Stretching Practice

Creating a supportive environment for regular stretching practice can help you stay motivated and committed to your routine.

Here are some suggestions for creating an environment that fosters regular stretching practice:

1. Designate a Stretching Space: Set aside a dedicated space in your home where you can comfortably practice stretching without distractions. Choose a quiet, well-lit area with enough room to move freely and comfortably.
2. Gather Your Equipment: Keep any equipment you need for stretching, such as yoga mats, blocks, straps, or towels, easily accessible in your stretching space. Having everything you need on hand will make it easier to stick to your routine.
3. Set Realistic Goals: Set realistic and achievable goals for your stretching practice, such as stretching for 10 minutes

every day or increasing your flexibility by a certain amount within a specified time frame. Breaking your goals down into smaller, manageable tasks can help you stay motivated and track your progress.

4. Find a Stretching Buddy: Find a friend, family member, or workout buddy who shares your interest in stretching and make a commitment to practice together regularly. Having someone to hold you accountable can help you stay on track and make stretching feel more enjoyable and social.

5. Reward Yourself: Reward yourself for sticking to your stretching routine and reaching your goals. Treat yourself to something special, such as a relaxing bath, a massage, or a healthy snack, as a way to celebrate your achievements and stay motivated.

6. Stay Positive and Flexible: Remember that progress takes time, and it's okay to have setbacks along the way. Stay positive and flexible in your approach to stretching, and don't be too hard on yourself if you miss a day or struggle with certain stretches. Every step you take towards improving your flexibility and mobility is a step in the right direction.

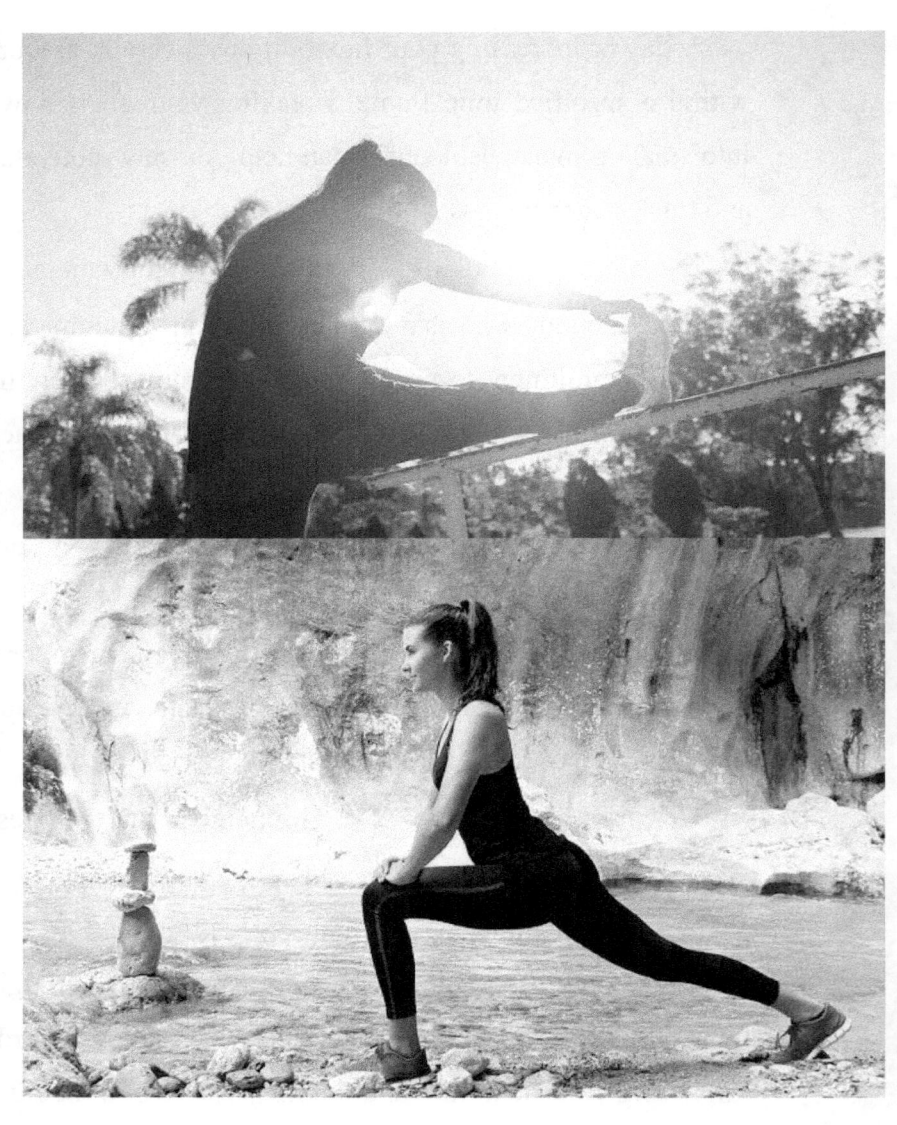

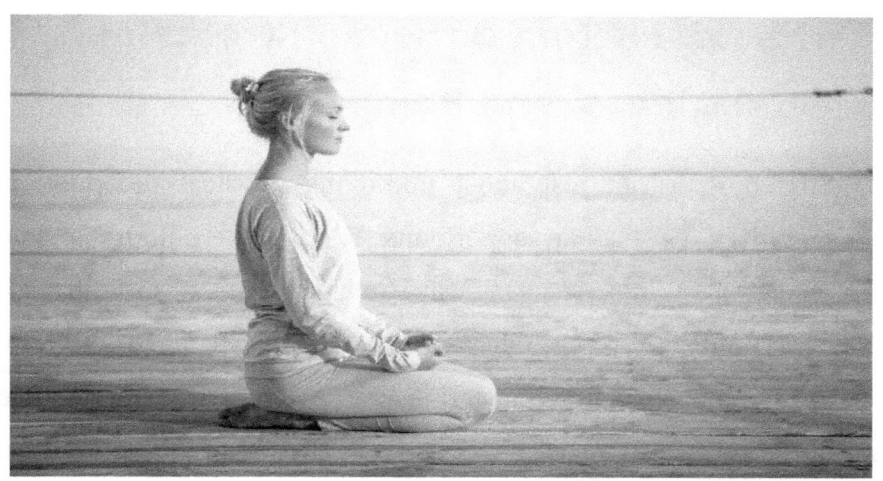

CHAPTER 8

Mindfulness and Relaxation Techniques

Welcome to Chapter 8 of In this chapter, we'll explore the connection between stretching, mindfulness, and relaxation, and introduce various techniques to help you cultivate a sense of presence, calm, and well-being during your stretching routine. From breathing exercises to meditation techniques, incorporating mindfulness and relaxation practices into your stretching routine can enhance your overall experience and bring a greater sense of balance and tranquility to your mind and body.

The Connection Between Stretching, Mindfulness, and Relaxation

Stretching is not just about improving physical flexibility and mobility; it's also an opportunity to cultivate mindfulness and relaxation. When we engage in stretching exercises, we have the opportunity to bring our full attention to the sensations and movements of our body, fostering a sense of presence and awareness in the present moment. By combining stretching with mindfulness and relaxation techniques, we can enhance the benefits of our practice and promote greater overall well-being.

Breathing Exercises

Breathing exercises are an excellent way to promote relaxation and reduce stress during stretching. By focusing on the rhythm and depth of your breath, you can calm your nervous system, quiet your mind, and deepen your connection to your body. Here are some simple breathing exercises to incorporate into your stretching routine:

1. Deep Belly Breathing: Sit or lie down in a comfortable position with your eyes closed. Place one hand on your abdomen and the other hand on your chest. Take a slow, deep breath in through your nose, feeling your abdomen rise as you fill your lungs with air. Exhale slowly through your mouth, feeling your abdomen fall. Repeat for several

breaths, focusing on the sensation of your breath moving in and out of your body.

2. Counted Breathing: Sit or stand in a comfortable position with your eyes closed. Inhale slowly and deeply through your nose for a count of four, then exhale slowly and completely through your mouth for a count of six. Repeat for several breaths, focusing on the rhythm of your breath and allowing each exhalation to release tension and stress from your body.

3. Alternate Nostril Breathing: Sit in a comfortable position with your spine straight and your shoulders relaxed. Close your right nostril with your right thumb and inhale deeply through your left nostril. Close your left nostril with your ring finger and exhale completely through your right nostril. Inhale through your right nostril, then close it with your thumb and exhale through your left nostril. Continue alternating nostrils for several breaths, focusing on the sensation of the breath moving in and out of each nostril.

Meditation Techniques

Meditation is another powerful tool for promoting relaxation and reducing stress during stretching. By practicing meditation, we can train our minds to become more focused, calm, and present, enhancing our ability to fully engage with our stretching routine. Here are some meditation techniques to try:

2. **Body Scan Meditation:** Lie down in a comfortable position with your eyes closed. Begin by bringing your awareness to your breath, noticing the rise and fall of your chest with each inhale and exhale. Then, slowly scan your body from head to toe, noticing any areas of tension or discomfort. As you breathe, imagine sending your breath to these areas, allowing them to soften and release with each exhale.

3. **Mindful Walking Meditation:** Take a short walk outdoors or indoors in a quiet, safe space. Pay attention to each step you take, noticing the sensation of your feet making contact with the ground. Notice the sights, sounds, and smells around you as you walk, allowing yourself to fully immerse in the present moment.

4. **Loving-Kindness Meditation:** Sit or lie down in a comfortable position with your eyes closed. Begin by bringing to mind someone you care about deeply, such as a loved one or a close friend. Repeat silently to yourself phrases such as "May you be happy, may you be healthy, may you be safe, may you be at ease." Continue to extend

these wishes of love and compassion to yourself, to others you know, and eventually to all beings everywhere.

Other Relaxation Practices

In addition to breathing exercises and meditation techniques, there are many other relaxation practices you can incorporate into your stretching routine to promote a sense of calm and well-being. These may include:

1. Progressive Muscle Relaxation: Tense and release each muscle group in your body, starting with your toes and working your way up to your head. Notice the sensation of tension melting away as you release each muscle, allowing yourself to sink deeper into relaxation.
2. Guided Imagery: Close your eyes and imagine yourself in a peaceful, serene setting, such as a beach, a forest, or a mountaintop. Visualize yourself surrounded by beauty and tranquility, and allow yourself to fully immerse in the sights, sounds, and sensations of this imaginary landscape.
3. Yoga Nidra: Also known as "yogic sleep," yoga nidra is a deeply relaxing practice that involves guided relaxation and visualization. Lie down in a comfortable position and listen to a yoga nidra recording or guide yourself through a series

of relaxation prompts, allowing yourself to enter a state of deep relaxation and rejuvenation.

The Mental Health Benefits of Mindfulness in Stretching Routines

Incorporating mindfulness and relaxation techniques into your stretching routine can offer numerous mental health benefits, including:

1. Stress Reduction: Mindfulness practices such as breathing exercises and meditation can help reduce stress levels by calming the nervous system and promoting a sense of relaxation and ease.

2. Improved Mood: Regular mindfulness practice has been shown to improve mood and emotional well-being, reducing symptoms of anxiety and depression and promoting a greater sense of happiness and contentment.

3. Enhanced Focus and Concentration: Mindfulness techniques can help sharpen your focus and concentration, allowing you to fully engage with your stretching routine and other activities in your daily life.

4. Better Sleep: Practicing mindfulness and relaxation techniques before bed can help promote better sleep by

calming the mind and body and reducing nighttime anxiety and stress.

5. Increased Self-Awareness: Mindfulness practices encourage self-reflection and self-awareness, helping you become more attuned to your thoughts, feelings, and bodily sensations.

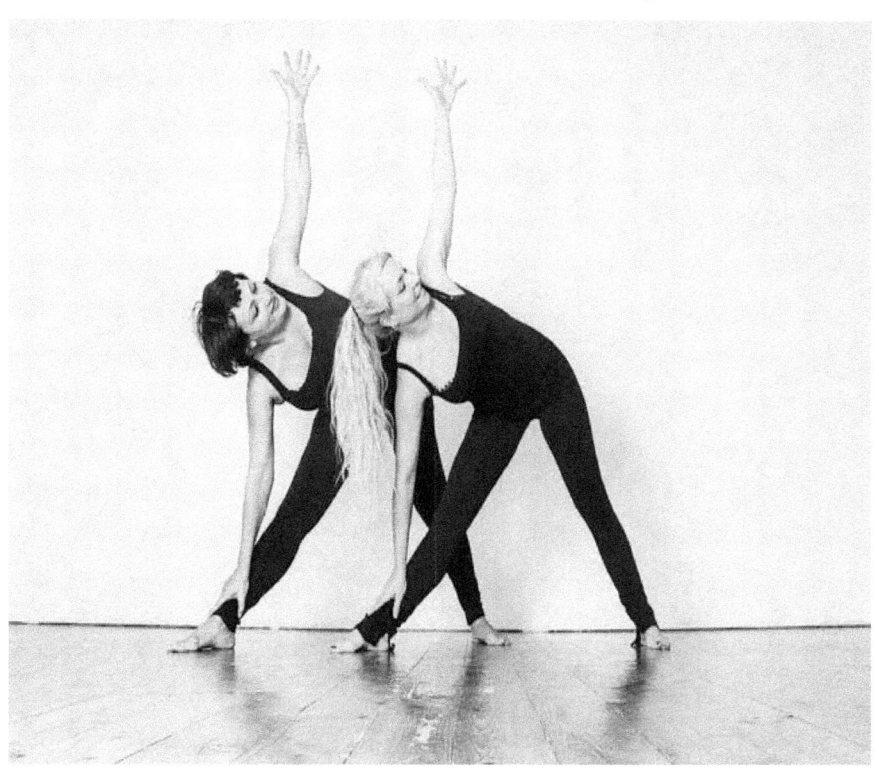

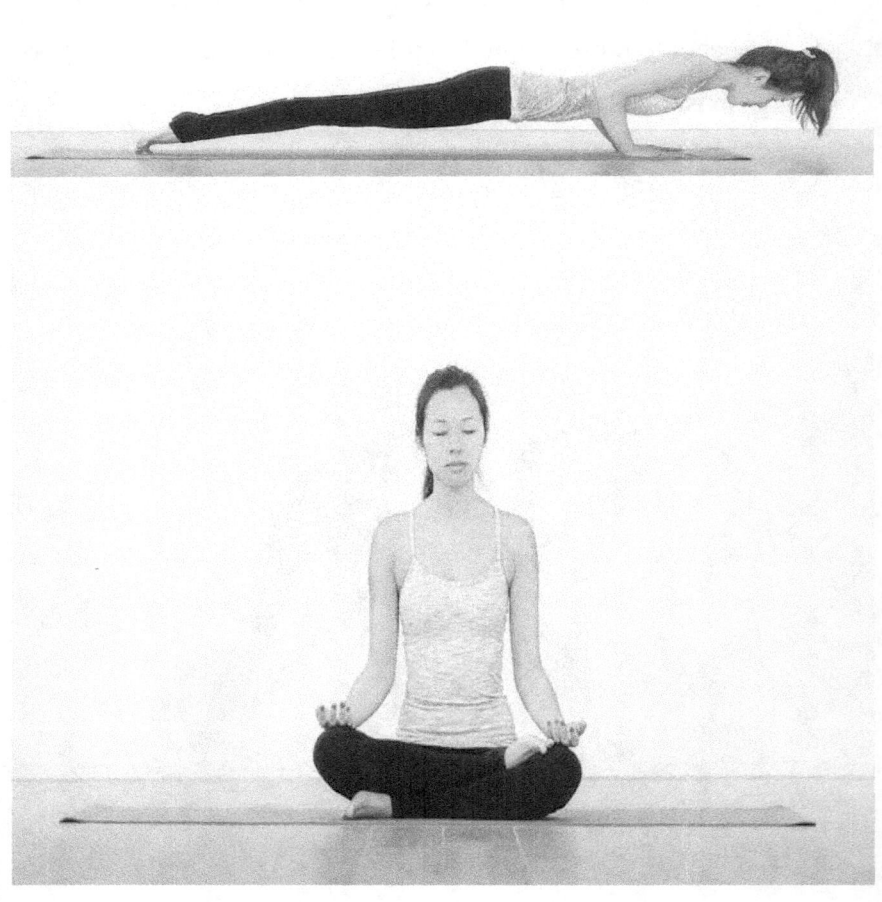

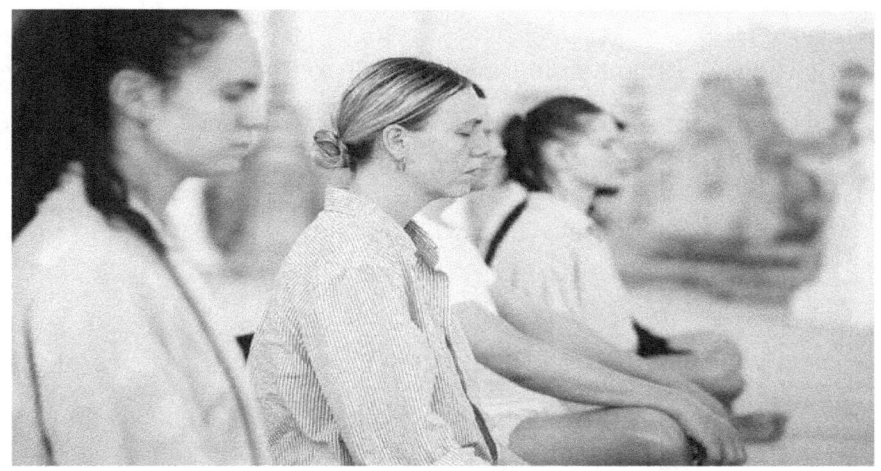

CHAPTER 9

Staying Motivated and Overcoming Challenges

Welcome to Chapter 9 In this chapter, we'll address common challenges seniors may face when establishing a stretching routine and offer strategies for staying motivated and overcoming obstacles such as boredom or lack of time. We'll also share success stories and testimonials from seniors who have benefited from regular stretching, providing inspiration and encouragement to help you stay committed to your stretching practice and achieve your health and wellness goals.

Common Challenges Seniors May Face

Starting and maintaining a stretching routine can be challenging, especially for seniors who may be dealing with physical limitations, health concerns, or other barriers to exercise. Some common challenges seniors may face when establishing a stretching routine include:

1. Physical Discomfort: Seniors may experience physical discomfort or pain when stretching, especially if they have existing joint stiffness, muscle tightness, or other mobility issues.

2. Lack of Motivation: Seniors may struggle to find the motivation to stick to a stretching routine, especially if they don't see immediate results or if they find stretching to be boring or repetitive.

3. Time Constraints: Seniors may feel like they don't have enough time to devote to stretching, especially if they have busy schedules or competing priorities.

4. Lack of Knowledge: Seniors may feel unsure about how to properly perform stretching exercises or which stretches are most beneficial for their specific needs and goals.

Strategies for Staying Motivated and Overcoming Challenges

While overcoming these challenges may seem daunting, there are several strategies you can use to stay motivated and committed to your stretching routine:

1. Set Realistic Goals: Start by setting realistic and achievable goals for your stretching routine, such as stretching for 10 minutes every day or improving your flexibility by a certain amount within a specified time frame. Break your goals down into smaller, manageable tasks, and celebrate your progress along the way.

2. What You Enjoy: Experiment with different types of stretching exercises and find what you enjoy the most. Whether it's yoga, Pilates, tai chi, or simple static stretches, choose activities that feel enjoyable and rewarding to you.

3. Mix It Up: Keep your stretching routine interesting and engaging by mixing up your exercises and trying new stretches regularly. Incorporate a variety of stretching techniques, such as static stretches, dynamic stretches, and foam rolling, to keep your routine fresh and challenging.

4. Stay Consistent: Consistency is key when it comes to stretching. Make a commitment to yourself to stick to your

stretching routine, even on days when you don't feel like it. Schedule your stretching sessions at the same time each day to make them a non-negotiable part of your routine.

5. Listen to Your Body: Pay attention to how your body feels during stretching and adjust your routine accordingly. If a stretch feels uncomfortable or painful, back off and try a gentler variation. Be patient with yourself and trust that progress takes time.

6. Incorporate Mindfulness: Practice mindfulness and relaxation techniques during your stretching routine to help quiet your mind and deepen your connection to your body. Focus on the sensations and movements of your body as you stretch, and allow yourself to fully immerse in the present moment.

Success Stories and Testimonials

To provide inspiration and encouragement, let's

hear from some seniors who have benefited from regular stretching:

1. Joan's Story: Before I started stretching regularly,
   I struggled with stiffness and pain in my joints, especially in my knees and hips. But after incorporating stretching into my daily routine, I've noticed a significant improvement in my flexibility and mobility. I feel more limber and agile than

ever before, and I'm able to enjoy activities like gardening and walking with ease."

2. Bill's Testimonial: As a lifelong athlete, I thought I knew everything there was to know about stretching. But as I've gotten older, I've realized the importance of incorporating gentle stretching into my routine to prevent injuries and maintain my flexibility. Stretching has helped me stay active and healthy, allowing me to continue doing the activities I love well into my golden years."

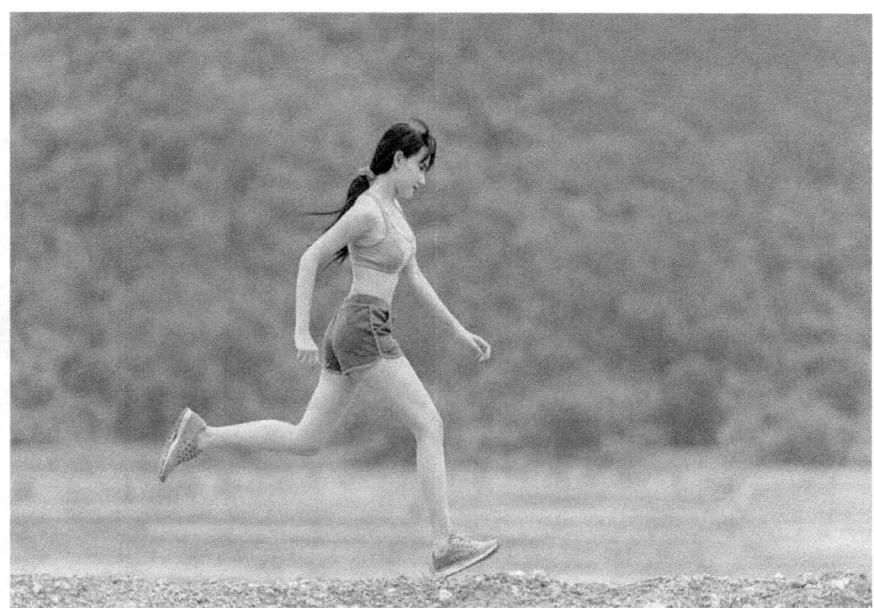

Conclusion

In conclusion, while establishing a stretching routine as a senior may present challenges, it's important to remember that with dedication, patience, and perseverance, you can overcome these obstacles and reap the numerous benefits of regular stretching. By setting realistic goals, finding activities you enjoy, staying consistent, and listening to your body, you can stay motivated and committed to your stretching routine for the long haul. And remember, you're not alone—there are many seniors who have successfully incorporated stretching into their lives and experienced positive changes in their health and well-being.

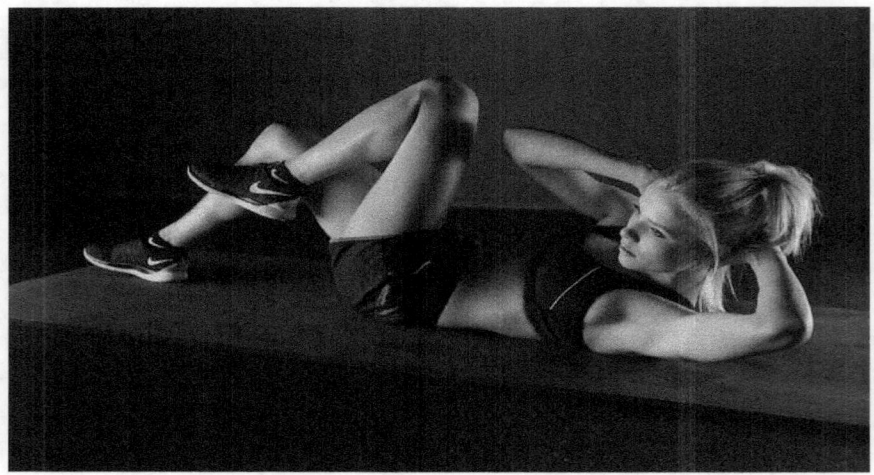

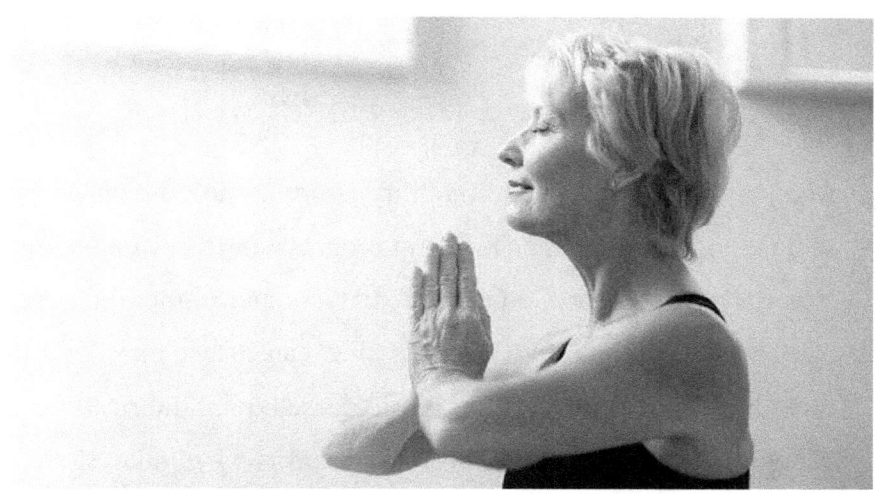

CHAPTER 10

Maintaining Long-Term Flexibility and Health

Welcome to the final chapter In this chapter, we'll discuss the importance of ongoing maintenance and progression in a stretching program, provide tips for adapting the stretching routine as seniors' needs change over time, and emphasize the role of stretching in supporting overall health and independence in later life. By committing to long-term flexibility and health, you can continue to enjoy a vibrant and active lifestyle well into your golden years.

The Importance of Ongoing Maintenance and Progression

Maintaining flexibility and mobility is not a one-time endeavor; it requires ongoing maintenance and progression to ensure continued benefits and prevent the onset of stiffness and immobility. As we age, our bodies undergo changes that can affect our flexibility, including loss of muscle mass, decreased joint lubrication, and changes in connective tissue. By incorporating regular stretching into your routine and gradually increasing the intensity and duration of your stretches over time, you can counteract these changes and maintain or even improve your flexibility as you age.

Tips for Adapting the Stretching Routine

As seniors' needs change over time, it's important to adapt the stretching routine to address new challenges and limitations.

Here are some tips for adapting the stretching routine as you age:

3. Listen to Your Body: Pay attention to how your body feels during stretching and adjust your routine accordingly. If you experience pain or discomfort, back off and try a gentler variation of the stretch. As you age, you may need to

modify certain stretches or avoid high-impact exercises that put excessive strain on your joints.

4. Focus on Functional Flexibility: As you age, focus on maintaining functional flexibility—the ability to perform everyday activities with ease and efficiency. Tailor your stretching routine to target the muscles and joints involved in activities you enjoy, such as walking, gardening, or playing with grandchildren.

4. Include Balance and Stability Exercises: Incorporate balance and stability exercises into your stretching routine to help prevent falls and maintain independence as you age. Exercises such as standing on one leg, walking heel-to-toe, or practicing yoga poses that challenge balance can help improve stability and coordination.

5. Stay Consistent: Consistency is key when it comes to maintaining long-term flexibility and health. Make stretching a regular part of your daily routine and prioritize it just like you would any other form of exercise or self-care activity.

6. Be Patient and Persistent: Remember that maintaining flexibility and mobility is a lifelong journey, and progress may be slow and gradual. Be patient with yourself and stay persistent in your efforts to maintain your flexibility and overall health.

The Role of Stretching in Supporting Overall Health and Independence

Stretching plays a crucial role in supporting overall health and independence in later life. By maintaining flexibility and mobility, you can continue to perform daily tasks with ease, participate in activities you enjoy, and maintain your independence for as long as possible. In addition to its physical benefits, stretching also offers numerous mental and emotional benefits, including stress reduction, improved mood, and increased mindfulness and relaxation.

Incorporating regular stretching into your routine can also help prevent injuries and reduce the risk of developing chronic conditions such as arthritis, osteoporosis, and cardiovascular disease. By keeping your muscles and joints flexible and supple, you can move with greater ease and confidence, reducing the likelihood of falls and accidents.

Conclusion

In conclusion, maintaining long-term flexibility and health is essential for enjoying a vibrant and active lifestyle as you age. By committing to regular stretching, adapting your routine as needed, and prioritizing your overall health and well-being, you can continue to thrive and live life to the fullest well into your golden years. Remember to listen to your body, stay consistent, and celebrate your progress along the way. With dedication and determination, you can maintain your flexibility, mobility, and independence for years to come.

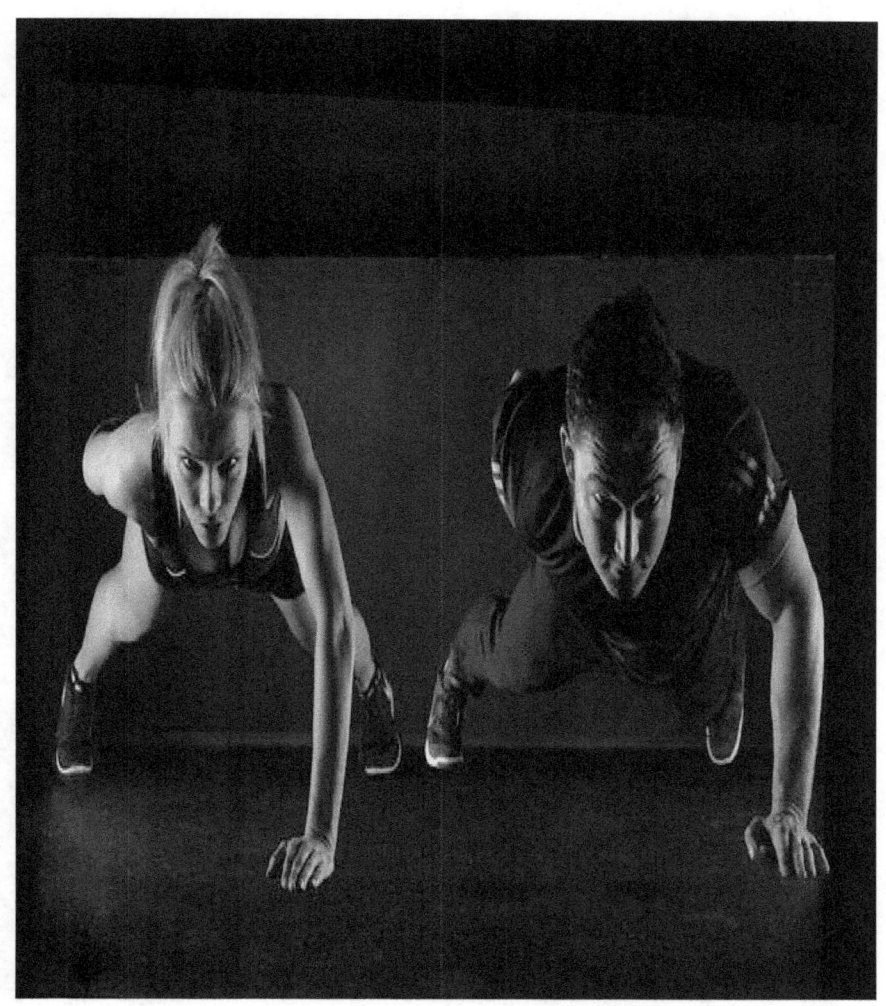

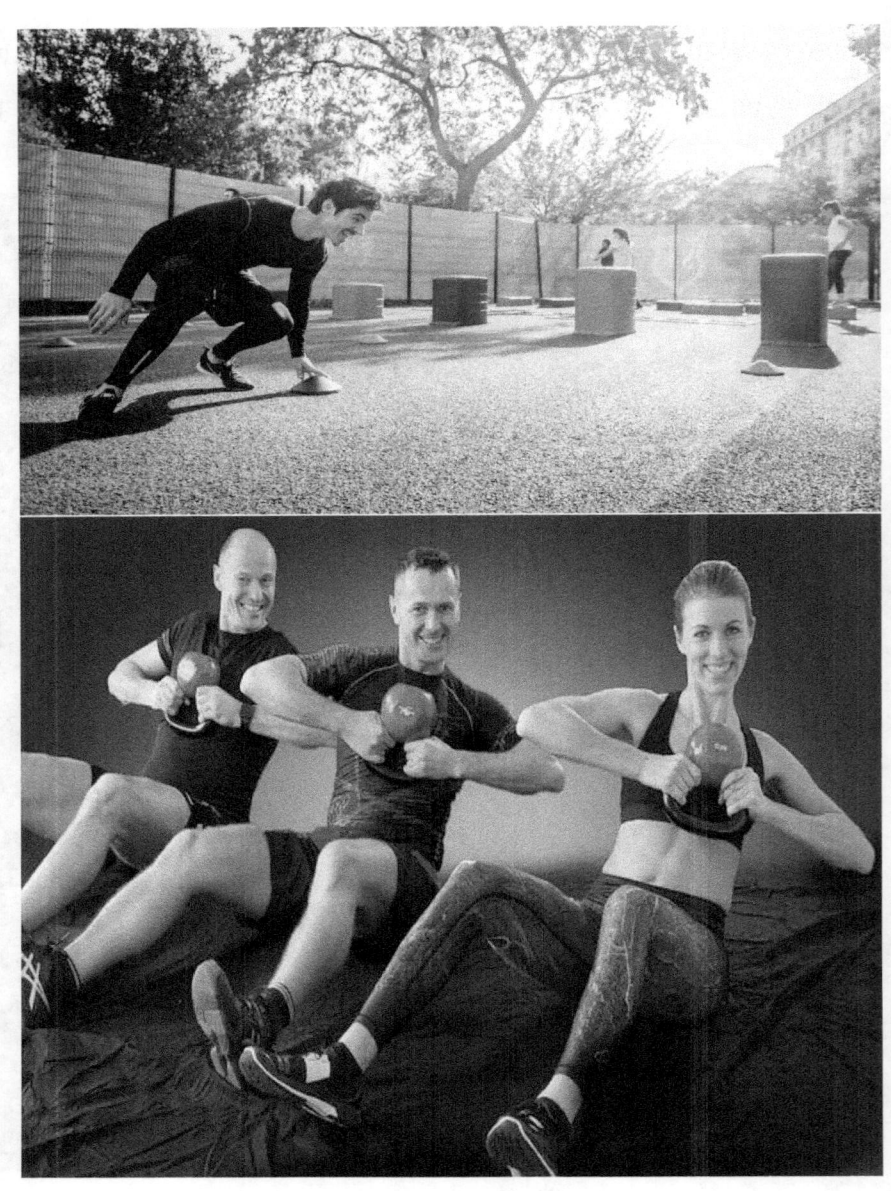

CONCLUSION

Embracing Your Journey to Vibrant Health

As you reach the end of "Gentle Stretching exercise for Seniors Over 60," it's time to reflect on the journey you've embarked upon—a journey toward vibrant health, increased flexibility, and enhanced well-being. Throughout this book, you've discovered the transformative power of gentle stretching exercises tailored specifically for seniors like you. You've learned how stretching can improve flexibility, mobility, and overall quality of life, allowing you to maintain independence and vitality as you age.

But this journey isn't just about physical exercise—it's about embracing a holistic approach to health and wellness that encompasses mind, body, and spirit. Along the way, you've explored the connection between stretching, mindfulness, and relaxation, discovering how cultivating a sense of presence and awareness can enhance the benefits of your stretching routine and bring greater peace and tranquility to your life.

You've also faced challenges and obstacles head-on, learning how to stay motivated and overcome setbacks with resilience and determination. Whether it's physical discomfort, lack of motivation, or time constraints, you've discovered strategies for staying on track and making your stretching routine a sustainable and enjoyable part of your daily life.

But perhaps most importantly, you've realized the profound impact that regular stretching can have on your overall health and well-being. By committing to long-term flexibility and health, you've taken proactive steps to prevent injuries, reduce the risk of chronic conditions, and maintain your independence for years to come. And as you've heard from others who have benefited from regular stretching, you know that you're not alone on this journey—there's a community of seniors just like you who are embracing the power of stretching to live life to the fullest.

As you close this chapter and continue your journey toward vibrant health, remember that the path forward is yours to chart. Listen to your body, honor your needs, and celebrate each step you take toward greater flexibility, mobility, and well-being. With dedication, patience, and perseverance, you can continue to thrive and flourish well into your golden years, embracing each day with vitality, grace, and gratitude.

Thank you for joining us on this journey. May your days be filled with joy, laughter, and the boundless possibilities that come from embracing a life of health, happiness, and vibrant living.

Wishing you all the best on your continued journey to vibrant health,

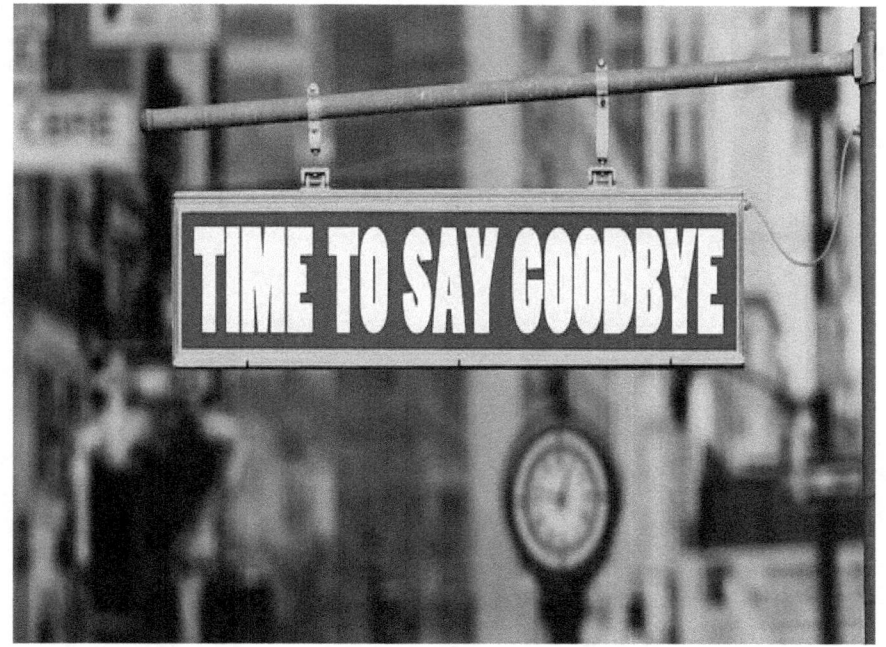

[BERNARD D NELSON]

www.ingramcontent.com/pod-product-compliance
Lightning Source LLC
Chambersburg PA
CBHW070401230526
45471CB00006B/2661